MW01712780

Dolphin & The Oracle

Authored by

Jean Charles Genet

Dolphin & The Oracle

Published by Thee Force Publishing
PO Box 283
Tavernier, FL 33070

• • •

This book is not intended to diagnose, prescribe, or treat any ailment, nor is it intended in any way as a replacement for medical consultation when needed. The author and publishers of this book do not guarantee the efficacy of any of the treatments and techniques herein described, and strongly suggest that at the first suspicion of any disease or disorder, the reader consult a physician.

Library of Congress Control Number: 2003096204
Thee Force Publishing / Genet, Jean Charles
Dolphin & The Oracle

ISBN 09626383-1-5
1. Health. 1. Science 2. Autism
3. Alzheimers 4. Chronic Fatigue
5. Debilitating Disorders 6. Dolphins Healing Powers

PREFACE

fic-tion/fik-shan/n. 1. Something (as a story) invented by the imagination. re-al-i-ty/n. 1. The totality of real things and events.

These two words, fiction and reality, describe *Dolphin & The Oracle* as the totality of real things and events in the form of an imaginary story. The way you interpret my story is dependent almost entirely on the events of your life and the unique way you view the world. In the minds of some, this could only be an imaginary story, for no one could experience such a life and live through it. Others will recognize the fabric of reality and be able to identify with the events and circumstances of my life. The label you attach to this book is far less important than the information contained within these pages, and my hope is that you will absorb this information and be able to incorporate it into your life. I can tell you that I believe this is a story of how the gods bring the right people together at the right time for the right reasons to achieve something greater than they could have by themselves, however tragic the circumstances that bring them together are.

Whenever anyone asks me about *Dolphin & The Oracle*, I always use the word "we" to describe all those who have in some way helped to write this book. "We" includes the spirit of wisdom of the guides and teachers of past generations who have chosen the dolphin as their voice; their guidance has been invaluable. "We" also includes those friends who have put up with the ups and downs of my life, those who will only remember me when I was down and would rather I stayed there and those who prefer me when I'm on top.

CHAPTER ONE

Autism Prism
Light Too Bright Cannot See
Me Right

I WAS THE SWIZZLE STICK IN THE DAIQUIRI OF LIFE

I was born in the heart of America in 1946. As each month of my young life went by, my parents took a moment to cautiously celebrate my determination to stay alive. Not a single month went by that I didn't face some new physical demon that threatened to rob me of my very existence. I was allergic to my mother's milk. I was anemic. At one point, a doctor confided to my mother that it seemed as if I was trying my best to get back to the Other Side. Little did my parents know how true that doctor's observation was.

Despite my apparent desire to leave the earth and return home, my parents remained determined that I should stay. They took me to endless doctors, and when I was four months old, I was given a DPT shot, an inoculation regularly given to babies to prevent diphtheria, pertussis or whooping cough, and tetanus, standard practice, except in my case. I developed what was thought at that time to be an allergic reaction to the pertussis portion of the vaccine, and within 24 hours I was suffering with grand mal seizures and exhibiting signs of autism.

In the 1940's the only method of bringing convulsions under control was to fill a bathtub with cold water and ice, and when the seizures began, to dunk the child in and out of the bone-chilling water until the child recovered. Little or no concern was given to the mental and physical processes an infant goes through when being dunked in and out of frozen water in the middle of a grand mal seizure. At that time all anyone knew was that drastic action was required to alleviate the suffering of a child who was having seizures.

From our perspective and knowledge today, we know that inaction is the best action to take in the event of a seizure, and that dunking a child in ice water in the midst of a seizure adds incredible stress to an already stressful situation. We also know that with each seizure I was literally dying, traveling back and forth to the Other Side. In fact, I'm confident that I would have stayed on the Other Side had it not been that the ice water shocked me and froze my vibrational ability to completely leave my physical body.

We believe that the act of leaving my body and crossing over to the Other Side some 3,000 times took me to a place of perfection where, over time, my autistic-like symptoms became less and less until eventually I was free from their debilitating hold on me.

I also developed a permanent memory deep within me and an ability to draw from that memory and cross over to the Other Side at will.

This ability has allowed me to travel back and forth, gathering information and perspective. I have seen that the earth is not the simple three-dimensional world we see every day. It is a living ball of energy with multiple dimensions, and when these other dimensions are accessed, our spiritual, mental, physical, emotional, and financial well-being improves dramatically. Unfortunately, most people have not had the opportunity to see the world from this perspective and there are those who still believe that the world is flat, with little room left for exploration.

I DIDN'T SPEAK UNTIL I WAS SIX AND THEN I STUTTERED

Ja Ja
Johnny Stutter My Words Again
Nothing Heard

A seizure is something like an electrical storm raging throughout the brain. It causes synapses to fire repeatedly and without meaning until the neurons are simply too exhausted to continue. This activity creates an altered reality and, in my case, caused me to enter a reality that produced symptoms of autism. I was cut off from the world, alone in a world of my own, and to make matters worse, the seizures interfered with the development of speech. Not only was I cut off from the world through autism, I was unable to communicate even if I wanted to. It took me six years to be able to form complete words and when I began to speak, I stuttered my name, Ja Ja Johnny. I began my schooling in 1951. There was not the clarity then that there is now about children with autistic-like symptoms.

In the particular part of the country where I was born there were no distinctions made to identify one ailment from another. There was only one "catch all" category that described my condition and that of similar disorders, "deaf & dumb." Being labeled "deaf & dumb" along with my strange way of speaking (stuttering), attracted children who were cruel at best and, at their best when they were cruel to me. I was the constant butt of their jokes and pranks, and when I demanded that they take it back, the situation only became worse; it took me so long to stutter out the words that I was only adding fuel to the fire. In my attempt to develop some kind of survival pattern, I quickly learned that it was easier to slug it out than try to reason with them. I never stuttered when I connected with my right cross.

I can now see that the taunting and abuse heaped on me by these children reinforced my feeling of inadequacy and fear of rejection, feelings we are all familiar with. When we are developing in the womb, we are safe and secure and all our needs are met instantly. When we are born we are rejected into a world where we are inadequate, unable to satisfy our needs and unable to function without the support of our parents.

These feelings of inadequacy and the fear of rejection created at birth are the foundation of all our problems. Being born perfect, then in an instant, having this perfection redefined as a negative projects the fear of rejection and inadequacy from all those who view you. I could only reflect back their fear, and in doing so, only made matters worse. My teachers feared that they were not capable of meeting my needs, so I reflected back their fear into what is known as "attention to task" skills. The brain of an autistic is moving at warp speed. The ability to slow down long enough to pay attention and focus on doing any one particular task, be it tieing one's shoe or, more in my case, reading, was virtually impossible to complete. The more fear my teachers projected, the greater my difficulty with bringing proper attention to the task at hand.

Fortunately for me, I had developed an ability to retain

information through auditory processes. If you could verbally explain to me what you were wanting me to learn, then the swiftness of the words being spoken kept up with the computer processing of my brain, and I was able to retain it. I failed at subjects that required little of me; subjects that engaged the brain to perform at higher and quicker levels I excelled in. Once teachers recognized this, they were able to challenge me with subjects that were not for the "deaf & dumb."

I graduated from high school with the hopes of continuing my education, but colleges were not willing to accommodate my particular needs. The reality was that the words "deaf & dumb" were still a part of my permanent record, and once again, the fear that was reflected from these words was predetermining the aspects of my future, which at this point, were dim at best.

Not wanting to give up, I sought the advice of those closest to me, my parents. My dad suggested that I do what he had done and enlist into one of the military services. This way I could continue my education and, hopefully, come out with a trade that would serve me in civilian life. I took his advice and enlisted. I was too naive to know that we were in the middle of a war where the words, "deaf & dumb" took on a whole new meaning.

JOHN WAYNE NEVER DIED

War No
More Killin' No More Pain
Just Insane

I landed in Da Nang, Vietnam in September of 1967. At this time the war had grown beyond our control or comprehension to a fevered pitch of suicidal proportions. The need to end the war was paramount, as it was destroying the very soul of America. I was oblivious to all of this because I had grown up in a state where there was one radio station, one television station, and one newspaper - all owned by the same man. Needless to say, my view of the world was his view and that was narrow at best. I believed what I heard and read, and John Wayne was my hero. He fought in all the wars and always came back to fight in the next one. My parents were in the Marine Corps following the depression. They joined in order to relieve the financial pressures of that time, and I felt that my only choice was to become a Marine like my parents and fight in the war like John Wayne.

As the plane touched down on the tarmac of the Da Nang airport, I was filled with a sense of patriotism with my parents and John, the Pilgrim, Wayne looking over my shoulder and pointing the way. My job was clear: I was going to eradicate the Communists from this foreign soil to make it safe for America; then I would return home to ticker tape parades, the respect of men, and the adoration of women. But this rose colored view of my mission would soon come to a screaming end.

THE NEED TO SURVIVE LEFT NO ROOM FOR PATRIOTISM

John Wayne
Where's He At His Hat
Cowboy Swagger

It was early evening in Da Nang when we landed. The pink sky reflected the tropical sunset as 124 other Marines and I cautiously departed from the Continental airliner. After 14 hours in the air, it felt good to be on solid ground again, and the kisses from the stewardesses gave us all a false sense of home and security. As I stepped away from the plane, the peaceful sunset was ripped in two as the sky exploded into balls of fire. The sound was deafening as I lay face down in the oil and fuel on the runway. Six minutes in-country and I was in the middle of my first mortar attack. When I felt safe enough to lift my head, I looked around, but John Wayne was nowhere to be found.

Rejected again, I would have to get through this on my own.I was assigned to a Marine Air Support Squadron as an electrician's tech, and since that job still had a live body working it, I instead found myself rescuing downed pilots stranded in countries they were not supposed to be in. It was a covert or secret operation that supported an even larger covert operation, and I was slap in the middle of it. The CIA was financing the staggering costs of the war with the export of opium out of that part of southeast Asia called "The Golden Triangle." The CIA humorously called their opium transportation "Air America."

Air America was the largest cargo airline in the world, and when their pilots went down, I would be sent to the crash site where I was lowered by cable from the belly of a helicopter to retrieve the pilot, destroy the plane and exit to a safe zone.

The feeling of hanging underneath a helicopter over a burning airplane is a surreal experience. I floated in a vortex of energy that was like the calm in the eye of a hurricane. While hanging from the cable connected to the bottom of the helicopter, all time and space dragged with my body as the only anchor to reality. Two weeks before my tour was over, while hanging under a helicopter over a crash site, all time and space were released in an instant.

Fallin' Down
Crash Site What A Sight
Nothing Right

I felt the tension of the cable give way, and I felt myself suspended, completely free for an instant. I looked up to the helicopter to see it autogirate, spinning out of control. The faces of the pilots and crew were distorted in pain and disbelief as their necks snapped. The helicopter had been hit by what, at the time, was thought to be enemy fire, and it was crashing down on top of the downed plane. Unfortunately, I was stuck in the middle.

NO TICKER TAPE PARADES - ONLY A CAST AND CRUTCHES

Johnny Stumbling
Marching Home Stand Up Straight
All Alone

The sensation of falling so quickly to the ground after being shot out of the sky is very much like being planted in a garden. Fortunately, the fuselage and exposed wing of the downed plane broke my fall and protected me from the full weight of the helicopter. I watched in horror as the chopper planted itself in the freshly prepared soil, recently plowed by the first crashed plane. Unfortunately, it planted itself directly on top of me, and I didn't see the light of day until I was plucked from this bloody garden four days later. Being trapped under that helicopter brought up memories of high school wrestling matches, and the sardonic grins on the contorted faces of the dead who spent four days staring down at me were a constant reminder that in this match, I had been pinned.

My rescue was like a dream. I was whisked from the jaws of death and transferred to a rehab unit. A series of X-rays revealed a spine not broken but stressed by a series of small fissure cracks. I was left with a spine like an old wooden bridge, ready to break at any moment. It would be years before it was determined that the crash contributed less to my spinal condition than a degenerative spinal disorder created at birth.

After I was checked into the rehab center, I found myself with boys who were never going to have their first date or play baseball again, and we were all at the mercy of the staff. I knew that the first thing I had to do was find a way to become mobile - not an easy task considering the condition I was in. In order to secure my spine, the doctors wrapped me in a body cast, much like the Pharaohs of ancient Egypt when they were prepared for their trip through space and time into the afterlife. My problem was not how to navigate the Nile but how to move myself through the space and time of the hospital hallways, and the solution was as unique as my condition. I was fitted with crutch-like braces on each arm. This allowed me to use my arms like legs to propel myself while lying flat on a gurney with wheels in a process that can only be compared to moving a tractor-trailer down a dark alley backwards without mirrors.

Physical movement in humans is a graceful but complicated process that is hardwired in the brain. We get up and cross the room without a second thought, yet the energy required to perform this unconscious act may use up to 90% of the brain's memory. This process can only be learned through constant practice during our early years as we continually reestablish the memory patterns and neural pathways associated with movement. As adults we reestablish and reinforce these pathways and memories all the time, but the doctors were concerned that the longer I spent in the body cast, the harder it would be for these memories to remain intact. In the case of movement, as with other cerebral functions, the key phrase is "use it or lose it." Somehow I needed to accelerate my healing process and unravel myself from the body cast before I became emotionally paralized as so many before me and lost the ability to take those magical steps out of the hospital. I couldn't have known at the time that my healing would come only after I volunteered to become a guinea pig for NASA.

THE ASTRONAUTS WERE GETTING AIRSICK WHILE ON THE GROUND

Space Jockys
Arrogant Bunch Lost Their Lunch
Flying Low

During weightless training the astronauts began to experience severe mental and emotional disorders that affected their physical performance. Western medicine which is divided into two parts, drugs and surgery, or as I like to call it, "body mechanics," was at a loss to solve this problem. Apparently, Western medicine goes upside down like the rest of us in a weightless environment. As you can imagine, NASA was frantic to find a solution and in a hurry. The race for space was at full steam. It was imperative that we beat the Russkies into space, and sick and confused astronauts were not any help. True to the American Way, if all else fails, find out what the competition is doing and copy it. The competition in this case was the Evil Red Power - the vodka-swilling Commies.

The Russians had been working on this problem for some time, as apparently, cosmonauts also become disoriented in a weightless condition. They decided that the best way to treat cosmonauts in space was to bring in people off the street to measure their response to, for instance, a pain killer. The response that could be measured consistently turned out to be brainwave frequency. When given a pain pill, the chemical makeup of the pill creates a certain brain frequency or vibration that when joined with existing chemicals in the brain, results in a harmonic (the joining of two or more frequencies together). This opens a door into the subconscious that the patient passes through into an area that is free of pain. The chemical in the pain killer resonates with existing brain chemicals to produce a reality that is pain free. This is important because the chemicals are combining to produce a certain brainwave frequency, and the recognition of that frequency is the important discovery. As the potency of the pain pill wears off, the patient moves back into the reality or frequency that originally harbored the pain. In essence, the use of the pain killer takes the user out of the reality of pain and into a reality that doesn't have pain. When this theory is expanded, we can see that anyone can move from a reality that contains a disorder into a reality that is free of the effects of that disorder. This insight was a major contribution to understanding the way drugs perform their magic in the brain, the way they manage different levels of awareness. An even greater contribution from this Russian research project was the ability to record each specific frequency that the brain moved into when free of pain or free of the effects of the disorder being studied. It's easy to see that the possibility of recreating the proper brainwave frequency that keeps one free of pain means you can bypass the need to use the drug, and this is a perfect solution for maintaining health in space. Cosmonauts could simply hook up to a machine that assisted their brains into the frequencies of health, and they remained healthy.

The problem, or one of the problems, was how to safely assist the brain in creating the proper brainwave frequency without frying the brain with too much juice. In an effort to solve the problem, the Russians developed a machine called the "Electro Sleep Machine." The machine created a mild current through a headband worn by the patient on the outside of the cranial case. This current passed through the cranium, and the brain received the preset frequency. For example, the frequency believed to create a reality that is free of stress and anxiety was sent through the headband and the patient's brain locked onto it and moved into that reality. This process is called "Cranial Electrical Stimulation" or CES. The process of electrical stimulation to enhance healing dates back to the Egyptians who would place an electric eel on an injured area. The French used CES in a mild electrical shock to the cranial case in the early 1900 's to address sleep disorders.

When NASA found out about the Russian research, they sought to develop their own Cranial Electrical Stimulator or what is also known as a Brain Entrainment Device. Without the original Russian research, test subjects would be needed in order to understand the dynamics and effects of CES. But NASA's astronauts were far too valuable, and hijacking people off the streets for their research was not an option. What they needed were subjects who were already under government control and who also had a variety of mental, emotional, and physical disorders. What luck! Vietnam was producing new test subjects every day!

THIS LITTLE PIGGY WENT WEE WEE WEE ALL THE WAY HOME

Bed Wheels
Crashing Left Crashing Right No
Way Out

Meanwhile back in the middle of the hospital hallway, I heard a new voice curse me.

"Hell, it won't work now," it said. "The frequency band will have to be adjusted."

"You crash into me and you're worried about some frickin' machine?"

"This 'machine' is an oscilloscope, you idiot!"

"What the hell is an oscilloscope?" I yelled, trying to roll over with about as much success as a turtle on its back.

"Doctors are using it to train idiots like you to walk," said the man.

There are no accidents in life. I immediately found a way to volunteer as a consultant and be a guinea pig for this project. I cared less about helping Uncle Sam and NASA find a way to treat some space jockeys who would float in a tin can above Mother Earth than I did about finding a way to facilitate my own treatment and walk out of this hospital on my own.

An oscilloscope is an instrument that displays the pattern of frequencies, especially brainwave frequencies. Since the technology to develop a brain entrainment device had not yet been developed, we (the guinea pig brigade) were shown the pattern of individual frequencies on the oscilloscope, told the purpose of that frequency and asked to duplicate it. A typical session involved sitting in front of the oscilloscope screen watching a wave pattern on the screen and being told, "You are moving into the reality free of stress and anxiety." Fortunately, my ability to access the Other Side prepared me from birth to develop a conscious memory of how these subtle realities felt, realities that are normally experienced only during the sleep cycle. If I could access these frequencies while awake, I could gain some form of control over my mental, emotional, and physical well being.

Every day I sat in front of the oscilloscope, opening my mind to receive the signal that would become the bridge between my mental and physical being. The medical staff offered no hope for this experimental therapy to actually work; in fact, their advice was that I should simply resolve myself to the fact that my inability to move might take longer than expected. They're still probably scratching their heads at the outcome.

HALLELUJAH! HALLELUJAH!
FREE AT LAST!

Cast Off
From The Shore of Pain
Happy Again

I never smelled anything as bad, even in all my experience pulling bodies out of the steaming jungles of southeast Asia. The inside of the cast had been attached to the outside of my body in such a way that I was discovering a whole new meaning of the word "stench." As the high pitched whine of the plaster saw cut through my cast, I was elated. No longer would I have to devise ingenious bends of coat hangers to scratch those hidden spots of irritation that drove me crazy. The nurses and doctors went about their business with a cool detachment.

"Now, you haven't moved in some time," said the doctor, "so don't be disappointed if there is no movement."

They had been preparing me for a riveting future since I first came in. My mind was racing nearly as fast as my heart. Tears began to spill over and roll down my cheeks. What if it was true? What if I couldn't move?

"He's moving! He's moving!" exclaimed one of the nurses.

The reason I was able to move after being immobile was my ability to access and enter a certain brainwave frequency that holds the memory for physical movement. I believe it is this frequency that opens the door to a reality where movement is certain. While in this reality the brain is able to maintain the memory of movement and retrain the body. My ability to enter other frequencies helped me sustain my mental, physical, emotional, and spiritual health.

Physical therapy before and after removal of the cast not only helped me maintain muscle elasticity, but also helped my body hold the memory of physical movement.

One of the responses to what we thought was my allergic reaction to the pertussis vaccine I received when I was four months old moved me into a reality where I stuttered my words. One of the side effects of CES training was the ability to move out of that reality and into a reality free of stuttering. I haven't stuttered once in the last 25 years.

CHAPTER TWO

Past Lives
Never Would Have Guessed The
Guru Who?

REDRESSED TO THE PAST

After my return to "the world," I moved to southern California to take advantage of the education programs paid for by the GI Bill. Since Vietnam was not a "declared war," I only had eight years to take advantage of these benefits. In comparison, my parents who were in the "declared" World War II, still have their benefits.

I decided to attend an eastern religions class which was being taught at a small community college, and as I discovered, there are no accidents in life. The instructor's love for music with a western flair attributed to our nickname for him: Hank (as in Williams) the Buddhist. My ability to play the guitar came in handy in developing a relationship with Hank and allowed me the opportunity to explore new levels of awareness that brought back memories of my many walks on the Other Side. In fact, my ability to describe the scenery on the Other Side gave Hank reason to probe deeper into my past.

"Have you ever been regressed?" he asked one day.

I looked at Hank through narrowed eyes, wondering what in the world he was talking about.

"Have I ever been redressed?" I asked.

"Not redressed," he chuckled. "Have you ever been regressed? Have you ever explored the possibility of past lives?"

"No," I said, "but I have always had a sense of being somewhere else before I was born." Hank just smiled.

The following week Hank and I went to visit one of his friends who was extremely skilled in the science of regression. He had me travel mentally to the Other Side into a previous lifetime. I remembered being in an underground room something like a basement but with adobe walls. A large window appeared across the top of the wall of this room, and I could sense the presence of a large number of people on the other side of the wall. I was dressed in robes as were the two other men who were standing next to me. I walked through an open door, up a set of stairs, and onto a platform. I was standing in front of a large group of people who were on the open ground before me. Behind them were two hills, and behind the hills was yet another hill. I seemed to be about to address these people, and I bowed to them. As I did, I zoomed out of my body, reinacting my passing over in my previous incarnation. I then passed out in front of Hank and his friend.

When I woke up Hank asked me, "Have you ever had your astrological chart done?"

"No," I said, rubbing my head and trying to recuperate. "I always go to the back page of the newspaper to find that information out."

Two weeks later I was presented with my astrological chart. I didn't understand anything about it, but in the center of the circle were several different triangles representing aspects between signs and houses. As I was studying the chart, the astrologer interrupted my concentration.

"Do you have any type of a mark on you that would be seen as a birth mark?" he asked.

These two were experts at confusing me; their questions seemed to come right out of left field.

"No, I don't think so," I said with a questioning twist to my face.

"You see this triangle on your chart here?" said the astrologer.

“Yes," I said, wondering when he was going to get to the point.

"Well, it matches the shape of a mark that is underneath your left arm."

"Listen, I would know if there was any mark under my arm, and I'm telling you that no such mark exists," I said with authority.

"Ok. Go over to that mirror on the wall and look for yourself."

I began unbuttoning my shirt and had worked myself out of the shirt's sleeves when I approached the mirror. Lifting my left arm up over my head, I moved closer to the mirror, and lo and behold, there was the triangular mark. I swear I had never seen it before. I was dumbfounded.

"So, is it there?" the astrologer asked.

"Yes," I sheepishly said. “But how did it get there? "

"That will be explained to you at a later time, but for now, you need to know that this mark will identify you to six spiritual enities that you will meet on the Other Side. The last time you were with them was some 26,000 years ago."

THE LAMAS OF LIGHT

Seven Lamas
No Humps Two Legs Robes
Astral Probes

Before, I was always able to choose when I would cross over to the Other Side. Now it seemed as though every night I would leave my body in the twilight of my sleep and travel on the seven colors of astral projection. I would first blast off on the color red, then merge into the color orange. The color yellow would become my steed and run across the astral sky with the color green overtaking my body. Blue would burn bright in the night sky of my mind as the deep purple of the color indigo would become a shooting star with pink explosions. I would emerge out of a violet sky and land on the Other Side. It was here that the Lamas of the Tje Jan first appeared in the same forms of light on which I had traveled to the Other Side.

I was levitating in space, nothing below me, nothing above. A beam of red, glowing, light materialized in front of me.

"I am the First Lama of the Tje Jan," he said as a pulsation of energy was emanating from his red glow. "I free the earth and its inhabitants of stress and anxiety."

As this experience was unfolding on the Other Side, I was completely at ease with the appearance of the Lamas, but I have to tell you that for some thirty years since the Lamas first appeared to me, I have felt very uncomfortable telling this story to others for fear that they would think that I made it up or that I was completely crazy.

Emerging out of the center of this red ball of energy, the Second Lama of the Tje Jan spoke. "I glow in the color orange, and I maintain physical wellness for the earth and the people that live on it."

Then a yellow brightness flowed out of the orange light and appeared before me. "I am the Third Lama of the Tje Jan. My duty is to enhance the performance and abundance of the earth and its inhabitants."

"What is Tje Jan?" I asked.

Radiating out of this yellow, pulsating, being came a green beam of light. The Fourth Lama had appeared. In a mesmerizing, low tone of voice, he clearly whispered, "Tje Jan is the essence from within of all reality. Tje Jan is the vibration of light that we travel on. Tje Jan is the frequency that wisdom travels to the earth on. Reality cannot exist without Tje Jan."

"I am the reality, free of physical and emotional pain," the Fourth Lama said. "Without the presence of Tje Jan, I would only be a vibration without spiritual force."

I was very drawn to the pulsating blue color of the Fifth Lama who stepped forward out of the green force of light and said, "Through my vibration is the longevity of life realized."

The Sixth Lama's indigo color was so deep that he seem to dissolve into the dark purple background of the universe's night sky that now overtook the vibration of the color green. He was the only one whose physical form was outlined in pinkish tones.

"I am the reality where you experience cellular regeneration free of disorder and the negative presence of age," he said.

Then the lamas formed a circle around me. My attention was drawn to the first lama. I began to feel an intense vibration of energy from this lama as his red light entered my pelvic bone and he said, "We are One." My body jolted as he disappeared into me.

As each lama merged into my being and said, "We are One," I felt more complete as a spiritual being. Once I had become One with all the lamas, I saw circles of red light emanating out from my pelvic bone. The color orange was emerging from a place between my pelvic bone and my navel. The color yellow was glowing out from my solar plexus and the color green was radiating out of my heart. Blue was pulsating through my throat. The color indigo was a beam of light coming out of my third eye.

I felt an intense pressure in the middle of the top of my head. Then a surge of energy shot from my pelvic bone all the way up my spine out through the roof of my head into a burst of violet light.

As I stood there gushing violet light into the cosmos, the collective voice of the lamas sounded through me saying,

"You complete this cosmic circle of divine energy. You are the physical incarnation of the spiritual body of His Holiness ZshonZshneh, Seventh Lama of the Tje Jan, Protector of the Mandala of the Soul of the Universe. We are your guardians. We are your teachers. Through our efforts you will eventually become the Oracle or voice for His Holiness to the inhabitants of the earth. You will use the Mandala of the Soul of the Universe as a 'doorway' to the Other Side where all past conflicts will be resolved. This will insure the safe closure of the earth's regenerational cycle, a cycle that has taken some 26,000 years to complete."

"But why will my spiritual vibration be known as ZshonZshneh?" I asked rather hesitantly.

"We are born with certain mental, physical, and emotional vibrations. Your vibration connected you to your parents and all the events that happened up to the time you met us. The name you were given by your parents identifies this vibration. Now your vibration is different and the signature for this new vibration is ZshonZshneh."

"But how am I going to tell my parents and friends that I no longer have the name I was born with?" I said.

"Maybe you would be more comfortable with the physical vibrational sound of your spiritual name." said the Lama.

"And what would that name be?" I asked with some hestitation.

“The physical vibrational sound of ZshonZshneh is Jean Genet.”

“What kind of a name is Jean Genet?” I said with some arrogance in my voice.

“It is a name that you will gladly identify yourself with in the future for to be known otherwise could possibly get you killed," said the lama.

"Get me killed? Are you crazy?" I said with disbelief and anger.

"No. We are not crazy, but don't worry, you'll survive."

Suddenly I awoke in my own bed. I was physically vibrating with the mental vibrations of my new name Jean Genet.

"What an incredible dream! Did this really happen? No way!"

But, as with all dreams, the images of my dreams began to fade into the Other Side.

In my next dream I thought I was traveling to see Dolly, but instead I ran into the Dalai.

DALAI NOT DOLLY

Dolly's Dollies
Don't be confused Skin Tight
Spiritual Light

Soon after my experience with the lamas, I was invited by a friend, then an editor of a large West Coast newspaper, to go with him to see someone called Dalai. Growing up in the Midwest and watching Porter Waggoner and his partner on TV, I naively thought I was being taken to a concert to see Dolly, not Dalai, Parton. We traveled to a Stadium where 25,000 people had gathered to see what I thought was a country western concert.

"Wow!" I said to my friend, "Dolly has a great following." As my friend turned slowly with a look of disbelief, the crowd went wild. Dolly must have arrived.

A group of people poured out of one of the openings in the stadium through which the players usually run at gametime and proceeded to move along the line of greeters, of which I was one. Standing on tip toe to get a glimpse of Dolly, my attention was diverted when a man in a saffron robe separated himself from the crowd and moved toward me. My only thought was that I wished this man would move out of the way so I could get a good look at Dolly when she appeared. Instead, the man moved directly in front of me and bowed. I smiled and looked around, thinking that he must be mistaken with his gesture, but this man grabbed my hand and began to shake it vigorously. The crowd was stunned, and I was a little agitated. After all, I didn't want to miss Dolly, especially after driving so far, and this man was blocking my view. Finally he turned to one of the people around him and was handed something. Returning his attention to me, he moved forward and presented me with a bronze coin that had his image on one side and a sanskirt saying itched on the other side. I looked at his gift and said, "Thank you." I promply put the coin in my pants pocket. He bowed to me as I had bowed in my past life regression, and then he walked away.

I turned to my friend who was staring at me and said, "Where in the hell is Dolly Parton?"

"Where in the hell is Dolly Parton?" he said, with eyes bulging. "You idiot! You just shook the hand of the Dalai Lama."

"Dalai who?"

THE MANDALA OF THE SOUL OF THE UNIVERSE

Monk Appears
Asking for the Dalai's Coin
Buddha's Birth

Sometime after my encounter with the Dalai Lama, I heard a knock on the door. I opened the door to find some kind of monk standing in front of me with a package in his hands.

"You Jean Genet?"

"Yes, I'm Jean Genet."

"Lamas sent me. You have coin His Holiness gave you?"

"Coin - ugh - coin. Yes,I think I still have it." My mind was racing and finally landing on a five gallon water bottle that I put my change into.

"Why do you want the coin?" I said as my eyebrows were beginning to arch.

"You give me coin. I give you package."

"Ok," I said. "Just wait a minute," as I bolted for my bedroom.

There in the corner stood a five gallon water bottle filled half way up with my accumulated change. I grabbed it and began to lift it up, but it fell out of my hands with its weight, so I pushed it over on its side and inserted a ball point pen in an effort to dislodge the dam of coins. I pictured the monk shaking his head wondering why this idiot had been entrusted with this coin. A few minutes seemed like forever, but finally the coin came rushing out of the bottle. I grabbed it and pushed up from the carpet with my socked feet only to have them slip, causing me to slam back down onto the floor.

Finally finding my footing, I breathlessly moved toward the front door and presented the coin to the monk. He took it from my hand then inspected the etchings. A smile of relief appeared on his face as he said, "You Jean Genet." He then handed me the package, turned around and exited down the stairs.

Inside the package was a colored silk cloth peppered from edge to edge with white dots. I eventually learned that this was a rice stained mandala made by tying thousands of rice kernels on a white cloth, then dying the entire thing. The result is a colored background with a white dot design. With the mandala was a note from the Six Lamas explaining that the cloth was called the Mandala of the Soul of the Universe, and its most ancient of healing powers would, in time, bring the entire Universe out of darkness and into the light.

The amount of work required to accomplish this task is beyond my comprehension. At the time I received this treasure, it looked like a maroon and white polka dotted cloth to me, and I thought of it as a very nice gesture; then I put it into the bottom drawer of my dresser. As I think back on that act from my perspective today, I liken it to putting the Ark of the Covenant into a storage locker in Wichita, Kansas.

According to the Lamas, India brought this cloth with them when they introduced Buddhism into Tibet over 2,000 years ago. The Lamas tell stories about the future Buddha, Sidhartha, being born on this cloth. Most believe this is just folklore, although I find the Lamas' stories most convincing.

As I manifest each step of my own spiritual transformation, certain images on the Mandala change in color from white to green and then to gold. It's more than interesting to watch this Mandala grow and evolve. Images that were hidden from my eyes suddenly make themselves known, as if reminding me of the wording of the note from the Lamas that the patterns of the Mandala are moving out of darkness and into light.

Now in the twilight of my sleep, the Lamas began to use their individual colors to download their teachings into my being. Once complete, the energy of this wisdom would draw me to people and events that would test my values and integrity as to the proper use of this wisdom.

As long as I held fast to my values and integrity, I passed what the Lamas called an "Initiation" and I would go through the same process time and again but at a higher level of vibration and intensity. For me to become an Oracle or voice to the world, the Lamas believed that I needed to experience all the trials and tribulations that define who we are.

Little did I know, the pain and suffering I would have to go through to define myself as a spiritual being in a physical body would be dramatic.

HAPPY TRAILS TO YOU

Concert Mess
No Gas No Show Only
Money Woes

After soaking up as many eastern religion courses as I possibly could, I yearned to find a way to serve. I continued to have the visions that were triggered by my past-life regression. In the moments before I fell asleep, I would see a large meadow filled with people, much like the scene I remembered from my past life, only this time I was in the audience. There was a band on stage, and tents outlined the meadow with dozens of sideshows of activity. And always a cool presence of mountain air filled my vision. Before the year was out, I found myself in Colorado standing in the same meadow. I had decided to put on the first environmental rock concert, and this was to be the spot. Unfortunately, I appeared in Colorado about the same time that Governor Love was vowing to his constituents that no long-hair hippie freak would blast the serene environment of Colorado with, and I quote, "In-A-God-Da-Vel-Veeta." But that didn't stop me. In fact, I was inspired.

For the next year I worked with every office and official that could charge me for any possible permit, making sure to cross all the "t's" and dot all the "i's." I worked with local and national environmental groups and organizations. I cajoled and convinced agents and the like to arrange for some of the biggest names in rock to appear. Representatives of the Who, the Grateful Dead and the

Rolling Stones all agreed to show up for a Fourth of July weekend with a planned 350,000 long-hair hippie freaks.

We planned a city under canvas, complete with tents for housing, hospital, emergency services, fire and police, and shopping. We arranged for roadways, bus and air transportation, and of course, the entertainment complex.

It looked like the event would sell out, concessions were licensed, and rock and roll acts were booked, when the government threw a wrench into the works. In an effort to convince the American public the only way we would ever meet our growing petroleum needs was to slash and rape the Alaskan tundra, they decided to shut off all the gas pumps over the Fourth of July weekend.

Needless to say, Governor Love's prediction came true. No long hair hippie freaks blasted the serene environment of Colorado with "In-A-God-Da-Vel-Veeta." The next day I returned four and a half million dollars in ticket sales, concessions, and entertainment deposits.

I couldn't figure out why the Lamas would set something like this up to occur then pull the rug out from underneath me. I needed some answers.

THE LAMAS HOLD COURT

Lama Drama
Passed The Test I Guess
Now What

I was restless. I tossed and turned like a salad in bed. My ears began to ring in a high pitched tone. This tone seemed to be emanating from behind my eyes. Then it felt like someone inside my head opened up the shutters that before had blocked my third eye from seeing out. This tone moved out from my third eye and began to materialize into a physical presence. A pair of feet began to take form as if being downloaded in digital dots of energy. Once complete, the lower legs appeared. All the while the tone of energy was becoming louder with each manifestation. The hips began to take form, then the stomach, chest, shoulders, arms, and hands. I had a sense that the neck and head were complete, but the light was too bright for me to see any personal features.

"You question the outcome of your last Initiation?" was the response from this glowing Lama in front of me, although I don't remember physically hearing him speak.

I should have been paralyzed with fear, but there was a sense of calm pervading my bedroom.

"Since you brought it up," I said. "why would you have me act on a dream that manifested into reality to only take it away from me in the end?"

"Dreams," said the Lama, "connect you to hidden talents that once acted upon, prepare you for something greater to happen."

"Are you saying that all of this was just an exercise to prepare me for some future event?" These words were flowing out of my mind not my mouth.

"You sound like you don't believe you were successful."

"I know I wasn't successful," I said. "I failed when the concert was canceled."

"But your test wasn't whether the concert was held or not. Your test was standing up to your values and integrity in being sincere in your need to provide such an event, co-ordinating the myriad of people, agencies, purveyors, and entertainers in such a way as to instill trust in your ability to actually pull it off, and most important, your ability to rise above the herd and pay back millions of dollars to those to whom you could just as easily have walked away from. You are successful due to the fact that you passed a very important Initiation. "

I thought in my mind that this future better happen sooner than later, for I had had about as much fun as I could stand.

"I heard that," said the Lama. "and yes, your next adventure will happen sooner than you might like." I had better be careful with my thoughts.

CHAPTER THREE

White Hat
Trust Me You Can't Catch
Me Sorry

THIS LAND IS YOUR LAND

Building a tent city for 350,000 people was quite an accomplishment. In fact, nothing that large had been built before or since. New innovations were developed and tested there that brought the idea of alternative power sources such as passive solar, solar transfer collectors, reflective surfaces, and waste and compost recycling to the forefront. It was a thrill to be a part of the development, but it was more exciting to see these ideas put into actual use; it's great to know these things, but they're useless unless put into practice.

One Sunday morning I had a moment of tremendous insight. It was as if a switch had been flipped, and as we now know, the Lamas were responsible for flipping that switch. I began looking through the classified ads, something I never do, and came across an ad that read, "Rocky Mountain Property For Sale." What a coincidence! Here was an opportunity to put to work some of the knowledge of alternative power sources I had learned. I could finally provide service to others with the knowledge I had gained while building that huge tent city. I called my company Environmental Systems, and its purpose was to help people purchase property and over time, install certain energy saving and alternative energy devices so that their property would eventually function as an environmental system. The timing was right with the energy crisis in full bloom. The program was a huge success, so successful, in fact, I created Inter-Continental Land Bank to finance it. Then the land sharks began to smell blood.

Land sharks are individuals who are always and forever professing their trustworthiness and reliability, and to prove it they usually wear some kind of white hat. As you're paying attention to the white hat, they're doing their best to plow you under. The bad news is the land sharks are everywhere; the good news is they always end up charging more and more until they kill the goose that laid the golden egg. So it happened with Environmental Systems. The land sharks began charging so much for the land that eventually the price of the property outweighed the cost of development. Soon they were feeding on the carcass and complaining there was no meat left on the bones. Soon after, another Lama appeared much the same way as before.

"So, how did you like the outcome of this, your future event?"

"The only saving grace this time is that I didn't wind up flat broke like I did before."

"Let's set the money aside for a moment," said the Lama. "Do you know how incredible it is for you to take the knowledge acquired from developing a site where 350,000 people could gather to creating an environmental systemwhere these same people can live in harmony with the earth?"

"I know it is quite a feat, but I have to tell you that success seems to be fleeting at best."

"You will learn over time that success resides in every minute of every day. Before you will able to experience such success, you are going to have to pass even more Initiations."

And with that response, the Lama disappeared out of my mind's eye once again.

NEVER SAY NEVER

Not Again
Another Pain in the Neck
A Wreck

In 1979 I was sitting on top of the world as I knew it. I was in the process of retiring from the land business with a sizeable amount of cash in hand. I had just married Kimberly. Life couldn't be better, or so I thought.

I turned over in bed, heard something snap in my spine, and felt a warm sensation ooze all the way down my back. My neck had collapsed, and once again I was unable to move. Unknown to anyone including me, I had been born with a degenerative spine. Some think that this might have been connected to my allergic reaction to the DPT inoculation, but we found out later that this was not the case.

Apparently, as I grew up, my spine grew in length but very little in circumference. The combination of contact sports, fighting for my dignity through school, having a helicopter chase me to the ground, and yoga headstands finally took their toll; my spine collapsed from all the wear and tear.

I sent my records to the top neurosurgeons in the world and asked one question: If this were your spine, to whom would you go? Their response was unanimous. The doctor all the doctors trusted was in California. He had received his training at the same type of rehabilitation center where I had recovered from my close encounter with the helicopter. Once again, there are no accidents! I made an appointment; he agreed to take my case, and before I knew it, I was being rolled into the operating room.

The surgical team entered through the front of my throat because they wanted to approach my spine slowly and carefully. Lasers were used to dislodge the splinters and broken fragments from around my spine. Bone pulp was extracted from my hip and meticulously molded to fit around my spinal cord, and the talented hands of the surgeon recreated my broken spine to its original dimensions. "Original dimensions" is a key phrase and the key to the success of the surgery. The surgical team didn't leave very much room for my spinal cord to expand; every time it expanded in the narrow channel, it touched the sides of the spinal column and short circuited. The result was temporary paralysis in various body parts, depending on where it touched. On any particular day, I might not be able to move different parts of my upper body, my arm, or fingers, neck, or... you get the idea. In an eerie twist, I could usually feel this paralysis coming before it happened, but I never knew where it would strike or how long it would last.

Events like this have a way of changing the course of a person's life, and I was no exception. My retirement plans were considerably accelerated, and my new marriage was annulled. Having been through this kind of healing process once before, I understood the kind of difficulties involved, and I never wanted to put my new bride through this. Also I knew that I would be better able to work on the reconstructive process if I was alone and focusing on the healing process exclusively. I did not count on the depth of emotional pain this decision would cost me.

WATER, WATER EVERYWHERE AND NOT A DROP TO DRINK

Float Away
From the Pain Lilly's Dream
Dolphin Team

One evening as I was walking along an ocean front boardwalk with an old friend, I felt the familiar warning signs of paralysis coming on. The damp air blowing in off the sea was evidently antagonizing my situation, and I needed to relieve the pressure on my back as soon as possible. We entered a movie theater, bought tickets to whatever was playing, and went in so I could get off my feet. As luck would have it, the movie was *Altered States*, the story of one man's exploration into the deep crevices of inner space. The subject on the screen used a peculiar technique for achieving an altered state of consciousness, and I couldn't believe my eyes. I was spellbound as the solution to my ticket to altered states involved floating in a sensory deprivation tank.

I stood up in the theatre and yelled, "This is it! This is the answer!"

My embarrassed friend pulled me back into my seat, but I could hardly contain myself. The greatest obstacle to my healing process was the force of gravity pushing on my damaged and fragile spine. Anything I did to relieve my situation was immediately undone as soon as I stood up and walked anywhere. If I could float in salt water like the actor in the movie, I might have a chance at recovery. I couldn't wait to get home and get to work on my plan.

I was far too excited at the time to consider the incredible synchronisity of that evening. The chances of being in that situation, in that location, in front of that theatre when that movie was playing are astronomical. An event like that could never be duplicated without the influence of divine guidance. Looking back from my vantage point today, I can see that the Lamas were weaving their magic web, orchestrating the events of that evening into another Initiation.

The next day I contacted Warner Brothers Studio and found out that the movie *Altered States* depicted the life and work of a man named John C. Lilly. I resolved to contact Dr. Lilly as soon as possible to arrange the building of my own flotation tank. But where could I find him? And what kind of man was he? My curiosity was aroused.

I went to the library to research Dr. Lilly and found out that his exploration into the behavior of the dolphin is the key that unlocked his development of the flotation tank. Early in his career, Dr. Lilly posed a question: How does the dolphin send out a signal in a perfect sphere measuring two and a half miles across and decipher the returning vibrations to recreate a model of the seascape within this sphere in a three-dimensional hologram-like vision? Lilly discovered two consistent factors in the dolphin's ability to perform this miraculous task: first, the dolphins float in salt water which might facilitate the conduction of this signal, and second, the dolphins dive to a level where they are free from the interference of sight and sound.

I believe one of Dr. Lilly's greatest contributions was the ability to recognize that dolphins represent a higher evolutionary path, one humans can hope to achieve. With this understanding, he decided to create an environment similar to that of the dolphin in hopes of recreating the dolphin's experience. The sensory deprivation flotation tank is the result, and the experiences of those who have used these tanks prove his hypothesis. You must remember that at this time the medical community belived that if a human were deprived of all his/her senses for any length of time s/he would go crazy. On the contrary, when a person is immersed in a sensory deprivation tank virtually free of the influence of gravity, sight, sound, smell, and touch, the mind moves through multiple levels of creation. As embryos we were floating in a similar saline environment, and that is one of the requirements for our development into humans. In the flotation tank, the environment of the womb is recreated. I was ready to get in touch with Dr. Lilly.

When I finally talked with his office, I was told to contact Glen and Lee Perry of Samadhi Tanks who had flotation tanks ready for delivery. I immediately ordered a tank to be sent to Taos, New Mexico. By this time I had retired from Environmental Systems and had decided to move to New Mexico in order to set up a research facility with the purpose of exploring the process of brainwave management. This facility would eventually be known as the National Center for Intergrative Medicine. Little did I know, this move would lead me into an area of research that would forever change the way I handle mental, physical, emotional, financial, and spiritual problems. Instead of spending years searching for solutions, I could have them in seconds. But before I arrived in Taos, New Mexico, another Lama paid a visit.

"I know. Your going to tell me how well I did, once again, in passing another Intitation. " I felt that the Lamas may have gone too far this time in bringing about the collapse of my spine.

"I sense that you believe that we had something to do with the collapse of your spine. Is that correct?"

"Well, didn't you?" I said with a strong mental projection, since I never use my voice when communicating with the Lamas.

"No, not really. Unresolved conflicts from your past caused your spine to collapse. We did, however, use the event to test your ability to move past the possibility of being paralyzed and see yourself whole. Remember! Believing is seeing."

"Hold it. Let's go back to these unresolved conflicts. My spine collapsed due to the fact that my spine grew in length more than it did in circumference, thus causing it to eventually collapse."

"That might be the physical result, but there was a conflict with your parents that affected you physically with the fear of inadequacy back in 1492 that eventually took up so much energy that there was not enough energy left to support your spine, so it physically collapsed."

"I don't believe you," I said in angry mental vibrations.

"Well, some things are true whether you believe them or not, and we all are the sum total of our unresolved conflicts."

"Ok," I said. “Explain.”

"Where do you think our memories are held?" said the Lama.

"In our brain," I said with authority.

"Not really. We memorize much like a casette tape. There are thousands of magnetic particles on the tape, and the vibrations of whatever we are recording are imprinted onto this tape. Our magnetic particles are cells. Each cell generates 1.8 milliVolts of electromagnetic energy, and it is this energy that imprints our life’s experience. As an example, let's say you are driving, and you want to change lanes. You look in the rear view and side mirrors to see that it is safe to change lanes. You notice that a truck is behind you in the next lane, close enough to recognize but too far away to imprint your memory. So after you make your lane change, you will not remember anything about the truck being there. But let's say that you don't look to see if it is safe to change lanes, and in moving over you hit the truck. The impact will cause such a vibration of energy that a certain cluster of cells will be magnetically imprinted, and you will remember the accident forever. This is what happened when you had a conflict with your parents back in 1492. The energy of the conflict was so strong that it affected you physically, and every time you have new parents, this memory reappears, creating the fear of inadequacy, and in the process, affecting you negatively until finally in this lifetime, your spine physically collapsed."

"Ok. Hold it. You are saying that my memory is not held in my brain but in a cluster of cells that are imprinted with the vibrations of my life's experience, and that within that experience is a memory of a conflict with my parents that affected me physically to such an extent that every time I have new parents I feel inadequate, and that conflict caused my spine to collapse?"

"Yes, you are correct. I have to compliment you. You do absorb information very well when you are being spoken to."

"Thanks. Are you the only one who knows that this is the way we record memory?"

"No, your scientists are beginning to understand that the brain is much like a computer that doesn't store information as much as it accesses it."

"If our cells are imprinted with our memories, then is there anything like what, in computer jargon, we would call a hard drive?"

"Sure. Your hard drive is your soul. Whenever you die, you discard the physical body and take your soul or hard drive with you. Then when you are born again, you plug it back in. The doctor 'boots' it up or starts it again by slapping you on the fanny."

"Funny. My soul holds all of my memory. I thought the soul was some type of spirit that we carried with us from one life time to the next."

"In a way, yes, but in this spirit is held all your memories from the beginning of your existence till now, this very moment. How is your brain to know what to do unless it has a past memory to draw from? In your case, the brain processed the experience of your parents being present in your life. Your brain accesses the soul and asks it, 'Last time Jean experienced his parents, what did he do?' The soul receives the vibration of the question and matches it with a memory that is emanating the same vibration. The soul plays the memory in your mind which is the screen your brain projects this information onto, and the memory says, 'Last time we were here in front of our parents, we were affected physically with the fear of inadequacy.' Your brain doesn't know that it is wrong to feel this way; it only knows that you survived last time you were here, so it creates the same response again in this lifetime. As with any hard drive, memory takes up space, requiring more and more energy to hold its information, and after a while, when there is too much memory, there is not enough energy left for the brain to properly run our body's software, and we begin to break down mentally, physically, and emotionally."

"Wow. This makes sense. The question is, how do I get rid of the conflict with my parents so this memory won't be able to be played anymore?"

"We're not getting rid of the conflict as much as we are resetting its energy from a negative to a positive source of abundance so it can be working for you instead of against you as before," the Lama said.

"Ok. So back to my question. How do I change the energy of this conflict with my parents from a negative to a positive?"

"Your dynamic is not large enough at this time to hold all the energy present in this conflict, but at some point in the future, you will be able to reset this energy from a negative to a positve source of abundance."

"What dynamic?"

"As you pass each Intiation, the totality of the energy that made up this test is passed on to you. As this energy accumulates, your inner being or dynamic has to grow to accomodate it. At a particular time your dynamic or inner being will be larger than the conflict you are addressing, and you will be able to prevail."

"How big is this conflict anyway?"

"Let me put it this way. The conflict you have with your parents has played itself out some 4 billion, 936 million, 145 thousand, 222 times from the first time it appeared in 1492 until now."

"Hold it. No way. How could it have played itself out so many times?"

"Every time your brain senses that you are in front of your parents, every time you think about or experience your parents physically or emotionally, every time you dream about your parents or someone speaks about them, the memory of each event is held in your soul, and evidently since 1492, you have had your parents on your mind a lot."

"But my parents are my biggest supporters. They have given up a lot for me to have any life whatsoever."

"I'm not saying your parents are bad. I'm only saying that until you get to a point where your dynamic is large enough for your energy to be larger than this 4 billion plus units of negative memory, will it keep playing itself out in your life."

"Does this mean that every person on the face of this earth who cannot resolve their conflicts is doomed to a life of pain and suffering?"

"Jean, we all come to this earthly plane to resolve our conflicts. The problem is that when we are born, we are rejected from the secure environment into one in which we are inadequate to provide for our own needs. This creates what is known as the 'Two Great Fears' the fears of rejection and inadequacy. We employ the ego (who is this being who, vibrationally, is the sum total of everyone we have ever been) to protect us from the fear of rejection and inadequacy. Well, when we have conflict, it is either with a mate, family members, friends, or our profession or job. The conflict affects us spiritually, mentally, physically, emotionally, or financially with the fear of rejection or inadequacy. As soon as these 'Two Great Fears' emerge, the ego steps in and separates us from it, thinking that it will go away."

"The conflict doesn't go away. The vibration that makes up this conflict seeks out the same people that caused the conflict in the first place, and after awhile, there is enough memory to have this conflict play itself out time and time again. A life made up of unresolved conflict is called 'Purgatory.' "

"It is our hope as Lamas that when you become an Oracle or voice for His Holiness ZshonZshneh, he will be able to use your physical presence to resolve the conflicts that before had collectively doomed us all to a life of pain and suffering."

"When do you think that will be?" I asked tentatively.

"Oh, not for another fifteen years."

CHAPTER FOUR

Long Hair
Hippie Freak A Computer Geek
Brain Software

FREAKS EAT APPLES

Like most people, I travel through life making decisions about what to do next based on my past experiences and the avoidance of pain. Unlike many people, however, I am aware of the hands of the gods at work on occasion. I'm usually aware of this guidance after the fact, but sometimes I know as the events are unfolding. These are times when I do something completely out of my usual routine and I always smile and say, "The Lamas' Switch is being turned on again." When I arrived in Taos I felt the Switch go on, once more.

For some reason I felt compelled to buy an Apple II/64k computer. But I needed help peeling the Apple core.

Taos, New Mexico is a haven for outlaws, not criminals, but the kind of outlaws who are extremely talented - perhaps the best at what they do - but unable or unwilling to fit into the corporate mold. Fortunately, several computer outlaws roamed the prairie around Taos, and I found a long-hair hippie freak singing Colorado Governor Love's favorite song, In-A-God-Da-Vel-Veeta. This computer freak programmed space shots for NASA. We hit it off.

"One of the things you need to understand about computers," the LHHCF (long-hair hippie computer freak) said, "is that it works like our own brain. It will only give you back what you put into it."

"If I wanted to find out how the brain works," I asked, "could I use the computer as a model to work from?"

"Yes."

During this time it came to my attention that the government had disbanded its CES technology research that moved the patient out the reality of their disorder into the reality of wellness, leaving many researchers stranded. These researchers were invited to join me, and together create one voice to explore the practical applications of brainwave technology as it related to the perfection of health. This exploration would become one of the first models to train the medical profession in alternative ways of treatment. I decided to call our research facility the National Center for Integrative Medicine.

The next few months were spent breaking down the functions of the computer into their tiniest parts, then applying that information to structure our model of the brain. To push the envelope of creativity, we scheduled time in the flotation tank where great insights began to appear.

The first insight into the function of the brain is that it is habitual. The more the brain experiences something, the more it repeats our responses to it. For example, when humans first went into the jungle and crossed paths with a tiger, the brain recorded everything. The smells, sounds, colors, temperature, time of day, our accelerated heartbeat, fear, and our need to run or fight were all put on the hard drive. Now when humans go back to the jungle, the brain uses the same data (smell, sounds, colors, temperature, etc.) to find the correct neuronal pathway. We experience a programmed physical response based on what we have put into the brain, and the brain only gives back what we put in. Like the computer, the brain does not judge the event as good or bad, only that a certain response is required at this time, much like the conflict with my parents back in 1492 that the Lama talked about. This is extremely important to remember, especially as we begin to talk about health. When we are sick the brain records the environment in which we're sick . Then when we return to that environment , a room in our house, our car, our workplace, a certain smell, the brain accesses that tape and plays the whole thing, including the sickness as well as any other mental, physical, and emotional response. Before long the brain has created a habit of being sick, and it doesn't matter if you have a need to be sick that day or not. If the brain has created that habit, it will live out that sickness. This same subtle method of learned responses plays heavily into addiction traits, be it tobacco, alcohol, drugs, etc. Once the brain associates the activity of abuse with the environment, the person will continually repeat the pattern while in that environment. It could be a smoke-filled bar or somebody's living room.

Our next exploration showed us how to program our own internal computer to address our problems instantly.

BY PULLING THE TRIGGER YOU CAN ACCESS THE BRAIN'S POWER

Rainbow Colors
Coming From Space A Place
of Wisdom

Do you remember when you were going through a particularly trying time emotionally? Do you also remember that there was always some sappy love song, dripping with the same emotion you were feeling, playing on the radio? Even years later that song will bring back all the self-pity and depths of emotion you went through originally. Our research revealed that the tones or frequencies that make up the sound of that song join with the chemicals in the brain to create a harmonic, the joining together of two things to create a third thing. This harmonic allows the brain to access the tape and replay the memory.

The Lamas have a great saying: "Always solve your problems when they are small. That way you will have enough energy for a solution." Of course, Western society does just the opposite.

We're usually so out of tune with our inner processes that we don't even recognize the problems that have been festering for years. Again, problems exist because the brain associates the problem with the environment in which the problem occurs. Each time the environment is revisited, the brain reestablishes and recreates the problem until it becomes a habit. Over time we are the problem, and the only time we change is when the problem slaps us in the face one too many times and finally gets our attention. Then the pain of change becomes less than the pain of remaining the same. Once we recognize we have a problem, we have to understand the dynamics of what caused it. Then we have to search for solutions. This could, and usually does, take years, and I didn't have years to find the solution to my health problem.

But what if you could empower yourself to program your own computer with the information and feelings you wanted? What if you could program the mental, physical, emotional, financial, and spiritual performance of your choice, then create a trigger to access that behavior instantly and at will? The results would be phenomenal. Installing that information into your computer could be done by listening to CD's or through subliminal photography, but the problem would be creating the trigger to access the information or response.

From our example, we know a song will work as a trigger, but you would have to create a different song for each desired response. Smell is also a powerful trigger of memory. In fact, have you even been taken immediately back to a situation from your past, complete with sights and sounds and emotions, simply by smelling a familiar smell? How about the smell of pumpkin pie? Of evergreens? But, once again, creating a different smell for each response would be impractical. There was also the problem of bypassing the Reticular Activating System (RAS). This is a group of cells located in the brain stem that serves as your awareness knob. It is the part of the brain that makes you aware of possible danger, determines whether you might be harmed or not, and then takes appropriate action to run or fight. It is also the "Little Girl Who Cried Wolf" knob. If a message is repeated too often or too quickly, it disconnects the warning system and, in effect, turns the volume down. People living under airport approach lanes don't even hear the planes anymore, and people living next to stockyards don't smell a thing after awhile because of this group of cells.

I needed a trigger that would not affect the RAS.

I remember looking out my window at an early afternoon rain shower and watching the sun reflect off the rain drops, creating rainbows of colored light. I found my answer. Colors would be the perfect trigger because they have a frequency vibration that the brain already recognizes as a perfect harmonic (several frequencies combine to create the color), and colors do not activate the RAS. Each time a color is seen, the full power of the message is conveyed.

Of course, the colors I used to access the brain's computer were the same ones at which the Lamas vibrated to address stress and anxiety, physical wellness, enhanced performance, physical and emotional pain, longevity of life, cellular regeneration and spiritual wellness. I recorded inspirational dialog on tape that would enhance my healing, and every time I saw the colors, which was thousands of times every day, they triggered my brain and installed and reinforced the wisdom needed for healing. The response was immediate and continued to build upon itself by creating a new habit of healing.

Next we learn where the Sandman takes us and what magical doors he walks us through to regenerate us.

SANDMAN, SANDMAN, SEND ME MY DREAMS

Dream Team
Releasing The Disorder Of Today
Tomorrow's OK

When the Russians were exploring the subconscious frequencies the brain uses for mental, emotional, and spiritual regeneration, they also determined the path these frequencies use to connect and regenerate the physical body. This path is not a chemical or vibrational path in the usual terms; it is a pathway of time. This path is a seven hour period called the sleep cycle, and it's divided into two major sections in which we enter each of our four levels of awareness. The first three and one-half hours of the sleep cycle first involve a forty-five minute dive from the highest to the lowest frequencies. The next forty-five minutes move you through the frequencies again as you come back up the path and regenerate. During the second half of the sleep cycle, this dive is accomplished in twenty-seven minutes as is the return up through regeneration. These are the four levels of awareness: Beta, Alpha, Theta and Delta.

Our conscious state is known as the Beta state. The first level of our subconscious or sleep cycle is known as the Alpha state, the state which the brain uses to release stress and to heal physically. As we move deeper into the sleep cycle, we enter the Theta state where the brain establishes performance levels, adjusts sleep patterns, fine tunes pain control mechanisms, and polishes memory and the dream states. The deepest level is called the Delta state, and the brain uses this state to manage exhaustion, cellular controls, the immune state, and spirituality.

The most important process within these four levels of awareness is the dream state within the Theta level of consciousness. During this essential time the brain releases literally millions of bits of useless information from its memory bank or our soul. This is vital to our health because the brain records into cellular memory everything we do, smell, hear, touch, see, taste, and feel, as well as temperature, time of day, our thoughts, and the list goes on and on.

Our evolution has established a set period of the sleep cycle for dreaming. This dream cycle is approximately two hours long. It is the state the brain uses to access the soul and replay the events of the day recorded in cellular memory. As these memories are played, the brain makes decisions about the information that was stored in the soul. It stores the information in either long-term or short-term memory, plays out the information in the form of a dream, and releases the information. In a way, the brain cleans house during this critical time. Unfortunately, our world has become so busy, thanks in large part to the information explosion, that more information is stored than the brain can possibly process during the two hour dream cycle. We need something like three or three and one-half hours to clean the tape, but our biology hasn't caught up with our technology. If the brain cannot process the day's information, the remaining energy of this leftover information creates static energy or stress and disrupts the brain's ability to enter the proper frequencies for regeneration. The further out of frequency the brain moves, the more the brain creates symptoms to warn us of impending danger, much like the warning lights on the dashboard of a car.

As we are bombarded with more and more useless information through the newspaper, radio, television, work, etc., we begin to suffer more and more. Today, we take certain symptoms for granted, labeling them "stressful times in our life." We pay less and less attention to fitful sleep or insomnia, headaches, emotional outbursts, loss of memory, and mental and physical pain, yet these are all symptoms created by our floundering brains in an effort to get our attention. If we continue to neglect or deny them, these symptoms manifest into ailments then into full-blown mental, physical, emotional, and spiritual disorders.

If the brain can only regenerate and heal the body when it is in the right frequencies and the time spent in these frequencies is not enough, we're in trouble. And if the brain is missing these frequencies altogether because of the stress created from leftover, unprocessed information, it's no wonder we die so young. The human body is built to last forever, but we only live an average of 72 years. That's a mere 1% of our potential, and the reason we miss out on that final 99% is directly the result of the brain's inability to access and maintain the proper frequencies for a sufficient amount of time. My ability to access all seven frequencies for regeneration and to install the triggers for mental, physical, emotional, and spiritual healing through colors has brought full circle my ability to completely control the healing process and enhance my life expectancy greatly. This profound finding would be enough to have accomplished in any one lifetime, but I was soon to discover that in my topsy-turvy life, this was just the beginning.

CHAPTER FIVE

Rock Band
One Night Stand, So Grand
The Damed

MOSS GROWS SKINNY ON A ROLLIN' STONE

I had such positive healing results from using colors as psychological triggers that I began to look for a way to make this research available to the public. The answer came soon.

I decided to leave Taos and travel home to the Midwest to clear my mind. While I was there I had the opportunity to see the Capitol recording artists from Ann Arbor, Michigan, Bob Seger and The Silver Bullet Band in concert and meet some of the band members in the hotel lounge after the show. Our conversation eventually turned to my research, and I began to explain the process of turning negative emotions into positive responses. As we talked, I realized that entertainers appear in front of large audiences, singing about times that are more negative than positive: love lost, love gained, and all the turmoil in between. Every person in the audience listens to and internalizes the stories in the songs and begins to replay his/her own personal experience. This dynamic emotionally drains the performer, and no amount of applause can restore the emotional energy that has been lost. Often the performers have to be led off the stage to their dressing rooms still in a daze. The common misconception is that entertainers abuse substances (in whatever form) in order to escape reality. In fact, the opposite is true. The entertainer is trying to find a way back to reality.

I began to put two and two together and formed the opinion that entertainers could use my program for addressing their mental and emotional problems related to performing in front of live audiences.

As a benefit the entertainer's ability to regenerate, to immediately identify, understand, and find a solution to a problem, would change the entertainer's influence from pulling negative energy to giving positive energy back to the audience. This would put the entertainer in synch with a primary metaphysical law: One is stronger times the number of people positively affected times that number into infinity. I could see that entertainers would stop competing among themselves and begin competing within themselves, where they would find the right answers. They could literally begin to give more to their audiences than they were receiving from them.

I created Direct OnSite Care (D.O.C.) to help entertainers on world tours to address their conflicts. I used the seven regenerative colors to trigger certain understandings that allowed them to resolve their conflicts immediately. No longer did the entertainers or the production crew have stress overwhelm them due to the fact that the color red that moves the user in a reality free of stress and anxiety. No longer did the entertainers or crew experience physical fatigue because the color orange gave them a reality of physical wellness. Their performance was that much more dynamic on stage due to the fact that the color yellow was present in their environment. There were less emotional outbursts. Why? Because the color green was emanating a sense of well being. The color blue freed them of the appearance of old age and the color indigo enhanced their immune systems so they were less prone to getting sick. The color violet provided a spiritual oneness that embraced all of us on tour.

This same system of generating high levels of performance is now known as Mgmt 7 and is used with my clients after I have reset the energy of their conflicts from a negative to a positive source of abundance to maintain a high level of mental, physical, emotional, and financial performance in an atmosphere of spiritual wellness.

In the months that followed, I accompanied every top act in the entertainment business, implementing my research and indeed, changing negative emotions into positive responses. It was thrilling, but as exciting as it was, I was soon bone tired and needed a rest. The cold winter months were approaching - no time to be out on the road.

The experiences that were to follow would justify all the pain and suffering I had endured while immobile. The training I invented to keep me whole, mobile, and healthy would soon be verified in a way that would forever change my life.

FLIPPER CAME IN WEARING A SHARK SKIN SUIT

Dolphins Humans
So Much Alike We Descended
They Ascended

The sun was warming the blue waters off the Florida coast as I bobbed up and down in the gentle waves. Those long months out on the road were slowly melting out of my body, and I was enjoying the solitude and tranquillity. It had been too long since I had this much time to myself. Suddenly I felt a presence in the water. Immediately I felt myself being lowered into states of consciousness that I had only experienced during my early bouts with grand mal seizures and then during my time with NASA. I was mystified and I froze in the water, unable to move. In the distance I could see a large presence moving toward me, a single dorsal fin cutting the surface of the ocean. Remember that I grew up in the Midwest, and with limited experience swimming in large bodies of water, the first thing that came to mind was *Jaws*. My heart was racing; I thought I was shark bait for sure. Suddenly I felt something scraping my leg from behind. I still don't understand how I avoided a heart attack, but I turned awkwardly in the water to face my enemy. I wanted to look into the eyes of the beast that was about to eat me.

There before me was the biggest smile you could imagine. The dolphins had entered my life.

I immediately understood the inter-species

communication process between dolphins and humans. It was a simple process of the dolphins consciously generating brainwave frequencies to the human swimmer in such a way as to move the swimmer out of the reality of his or her pain and suffering into a reality of wellness.

My inter-species communications experience with the dolphins provided such an awakening of possibilities within me that I decided to retire from the entertainment business and devote my time and resources to developing a research model that would prove the healing effects of swimming with dolphins. Unfortunately, the G-Men got in the way.

CHAPTER SIX

The Cops
Stop, Shoot, Don't Get Caught
They're Bought

THE G-MEN ARE RESTLESS

The Drug Enforcement Administration or DEA (which we will call G-Men) was enacted to address the problems of drugs entering into the United States from foreign countries. The G-Men joined forces with local law enforcement agencies to combat this ever growing menace in our local communities, and laws were created to provide rules on how this game would be played out. The amount of funds allocated were determined by the number of busts or arrests made. The problem was that the threat of drugs infiltrating our schools and businesses was not as much of a problem as it was reported in the press. In government circles it is well known that if there is no problem there is no funding. Something had to be done to address the problem of the need to have a problem. Of course, it didn't take a rocket scientist to know that more busts created the idea that there actually was a problem, thus the need for more funding.

The first target was midnight Porsche drivers getting stopped with a dusty bottle of cocaine in their pocket. As a bonus a lot of these drivers had daytime jobs as highly paid sports stars whose services would be sorely missed if they landed in jail for any extended period of time. Plus the embarrassment of having one's photo on the front page instead of the sports page was proving to be the reason why the ball player was in a slump more times than not. Soon the word got around in the dugout that you might not want to be driving late at night with a substance in your pocket that was deemed illegal by the G-Men.

Of course, there are only so many big league sniffers driving Porches late at night, and soon the lack of a problem became the problem again.

WHAT TO DO NEXT?

Urban Assault
Wrong House Granny's Knittin
Dead Kittens

It was determined by the G-Men that there was a need to start a war on drugs. As with any war, there needed to be built an Urban Assault Vehicle (UAV) equipped with a battering ram to crash through designated crack houses. All major news organizations were invited to view this UAV in action. This massive vehicle was fired up, exhausts sounding more like jet blasts than simple fluttering of auto emissions, with the flak-jacketed driver sneering through his goggles. The clutch was released; the pedal was crammed to the metal, and this UAV was propelled by the driver over the curb, across the lawn and through the flower beds, crashing through the front of the house, finally resting safely in the back yard. Unfortunately, this suspected crack dealer turned out to be an 88 year old great grandmother knitting booties for her great grandchild. But what was even more troubling was that the UAV ran over and killed granny's cat.

All of these shenanigans were on the 11 o'clock news with side-bars of bereaved animal activists yelling at the injustice of killing this poor cat. Background shots showed the tire tracks imprinted on granny's body. It seem as though the war on drugs was about to end before it ever got started.

DRUGS, SEX, AND ROCK 'N' ROLL

Caught Drinkin
Search The Drunk The Trunk
Prison Bunk

In regrouping sessions, the G-Men began to look at those activities that promoted the use of drugs. The consensus was that those who enjoyed rock 'n' roll music and especially those who played rock 'n' roll music were probably the best targets to go after in what would become the New War on Drugs.

The New War on Drugs started at an alcohol/drug stop outside a Kiss concert. Although this kind of stop violated the privacy of citizens, it was deemed justifiable if the public was served when someone was actually caught in the possession of drugs or had drunk one too many beers. One such person, a production assistant, that I had financially assisted in retrieving her kids from her estranged husband, was caught with alcohol on her breath and four ounces of cocaine in her trunk. When searching through her purse, the G-Men found my business card. When asked who this person was, she replied that I had a company that addressed drug and alcohol problems in the entertainment business.

Before long I was brought before a grand jury investigating drug and alcohol abuse in the entertainment business. I was found in contempt of a grand jury investigation when I refused to turn over my personal records that related to my associations with entertainers. The G-Men's plan as I saw it was to intimidate me with the promise of ruin until I turned over my records.

PLAN - A..."High Power" -
Where Inmates and Rockers are all alike

Last Time
You Burnt The Toast Go
To Hell

After being booked, fingerprinted, photographed and dressed in County Orange, I was transported over to "High Power." This is the only place where guards are allowed to carry armed weapons. Why? The inmates are (innocent) people who woke up one morning to find their family members massacred because the wife had burnt the toast just one too many times. To the G-Men's way of thinking, being in this hostile environment would rock my world to such an extent that I would be yelling out client names through the bars in hopes that I could strike a deal before the inmates struck me. Unfortunately for the G-Men, fortunately for me, this scenario was not unlike being in the rock 'n' roll business. Rockers were just as crazy in their own way. They just hadn't been caught.

By next morning, I had sat down with my fellow inmates and resolved the conflicts that had led them to do such hideous acts. The G-Men were not amused.

PLAN - B Involved A Lot of Traveling and Fighting.

Crips Bloods
They're All the Same Blame
Bloody Cript

At this time county enforcement agencies charged the state an average of $65 per day to house an inmate. This became very profitable for the county due to the fact that it only cost a fraction of the $65 charged to actually house an inmate. The prison system became what is known as an "income generator." The prison system that I was assigned to was originally designed for 7,000 inmates. During the time I was incarcerated, this same prison held more than 20,000 inmates. When you multiply 20,000 inmates times $65 you come up with $1,300,000 dollars per day for this facility alone. The prison system was making more money in one day than all the hotels were making in a week.

By court order the prisons were required to reduce the prison population. This was accomplished by transporting one third of the prison population each day to a new facility. The guards would roust me out of my cell at 3:30 AM, lock me down with chains, and bus me to the next facility. I would arrive at the next prison around 10:00 AM. I would be deloused, given a HIV test, taken to another building that housed 125 Crips and Bloods (a commonly used term for gang members). Anyone new on the block would have the opportunity to become a slave for the dominant gang member. The only way to address this rather alarming set of events would be to remind this same dominant gang member with a right cross to the head that he had enough slaves, and the time for abolition had arrived. After 30 days of being on this road gang, the G-Men decided to bring me back into the County Jail.

PLAN - C...San Quentin Pop

Father Son
Rob Run Gun Death Jail
No Bail

Pop had spent his last 30 years in San Quentin Prison. The Parole Board finally believed that he had been rehabilitated when he told them that after 30 years of incarceration, he didn't care if they paroled him. Pop found himself back in a society in which he had no power. He had a thirty- something son that had tried to emulate him but without much success. Pop assessed his situation and decided that he needed to be back in San Quentin where he could reclaim his power. He enlisted his son in a robbery and, unfortunately, the person they robbed died of a heart attack. The District Attorney pledged that if reelected for another term, he would personally guarantee that these killers would be "drawn and quartered" then gassed to death.

To secure their case against San Quentin Pop and son, the District Attorney enlisted certain members of the prison population to be housed with Pop and his son in hopes that Pop would lament about the robbery. Well, Pop might have been born on Thursday but it was not last Thursday. Pop and son recognized the ploy and administered proper punishment to all those involved. The G-Men thought that Pop's form of punishment should be applied to me. Of course, I could circumvent this punishment if only I told them what they wanted to know.

During my time in the Marine Corps, I was trained to be a Golden Gloves boxer. Unbeknown to Pop and his son, I had been developing my pugilistic skills for the last thirty days and was not in the mood to be squeezed through the bars of the cell, which was what the G-Men said was going to happen to me. After round five, Pop and son decided that I was not an informant. I then began to put back their relationship. Pop recognized his unresolved conflicts as it related to his son, and the son realized that the need to emulate Pop's behavior would only lead to more trouble.

By now the G-Men were beginning to sweat bullets. If I didn't confess before long, they might find themselves in jail for their own illegal acts.

PLAN - D...Buzz Saw

Buzz Saw
Hell's Angel A Contract Killer
Death Thriller

Buzz Saw was in jail for being a contract killer for the Hells Angels. He also had developed a following in San Quentin and, like Pop, decided that he needed to return to the ole gang. Buzz Saw decided to rob a government building, and in doing so, got caught. Buzz wasn't upset that he got caught. He was upset because his accomplices turned States evidence. His solution...have them killed. No witnesses, no case. Once again the District Attorney enlisted cell mates from the general prison population but had few volunteers once they found out Buzz Saw's occupation. The G-Men were kind enough to offer me up as a roommate for Buzz Saw and informed me that right before I became Buzz's roommate his mother had died. In retaliation for offing the governments witnesses, Buzz was not allowed to attend his mother's funeral. Buzz was not a happy camper and told all who could hear that he was going to kill his next roommate. When I entered the cell, Buzz Saw was drawing satanic symbols on the wall. His eyes glazed as he looked at me.

My only response was, "Buzz Saw, your mother has a message for you. She said it wasn't your fault."

Well, Buzz broke down and began to cry. As so many times before, I took this tortured soul and gave it safe harbor.

Buzz got the message out through the grapevine that anyone who messed with me would be killed. This was alarming news to the G-Men. Nothing had worked to coerce me into providing them with information on my clients. Now if they messed with me, my friend Buzz was going to have them dusted from their existence as they knew it.

PLAN - E...The Hole

Darkness Prevails
Just Like Hell The Well
No End

The Hole is a hole in the bottom of most county jails, and this is where the G-Men put me to protect them from Buzz Saw. My hole was five feet by five feet. My nude body was eleven inches too long. There was a six-inch hole inside the five by five foot hole into which everything went and from which everything came, especially at night, whenever that was, for no light, I mean no light, was in The Hole. I could bring my fingers up to my eyes and not see them. Every day I was given a small bucket of water and a Jew Ball. A Jew Ball is a piece of rounded dough that, once folded, is the size of a hard baseball and contains cigarette butts, roaches, pieces of what seemed to be digested vegetables, and indefinable waste products.

Every two weeks I would be brought out of The Hole and taken to court. The cost of taking me round trip to court at that time was $185, a trip of less than a quarter of a mile. Being in total darkness for long periods of time causes your eyes to revoke the presence of any light. When outside on my way to court, my eyes, although closed, felt as though I was up against the sun. During court I was in front of another judge who was listening to another G-Man's story about how I had refused once again to give them the information requested, thus defying the grand jury. My punishment would be another loss of property, i.e. my home, cars, businesses, and of course, I would return to The Hole.

After a short period of time, I was more comfortable in The Hole than out in the light of day. Time is determined in the mind by the presence of light. Light equals day, and dark signifies night. In an environment absent of the presence of light, you do not know when the day begins and the day ends. One day runs into another. It becomes one continual day in total darkness. The need to keep your mind busy in a solitary environment is essential in the process of staying sane. Each day as I would wake up from sleep, I would begin exercising by pushing myself against the wall and doing knee bends. I would curl my arms forward and backward and stretch from side to side. I would then begin cleaning my cell by moving into a corner and using my fingers as brushes and sweeping toward the six-inch hole. Once my darkened cell was clean, I would wait for one of the Lamas to appear so we could begin our conversation.

"Boy, it is dark in here." With that said, the Lama vibrated into pure white light, illuminating my cell.

"Nice trick. How did you do that?" I mentally asked in a weak transmission.

"To answer your question I need to know how you view God."

"Its kind of hard to see God from this dark hole in the ground."

"I agree, but what I asked you is how do you view God?

“Do you view Him as this omnipotent being sitting on a throne throwing bolts of lightning down at us here on earth?"

"Yes. That is kind of the image I grew up with."

"Do you believe," said the Lama, "that this being is the creator of all things?"

"It does go along with the image of being omnipotent."

"All of us Lamas look at God not so much as this Almighty Being but more as a word that, when said, creates one of the highest vibrations we know of."

"How high is this vibration cycle?" I asked in my research voice.

"The ‘God sound’ vibrates over a 180 billion cycles a second."

"A human only vibrates consciously between 13 and 30 cycles per second of brain wave energy," I said, “and you’re having me believe that the vibration of the word 'God' is over 180 billion cycles per second."

"Well, He is God,” the Lama said matter of factly.

"Then you and the Lamas believe the vibration of the word 'God' gives life to all things?"

"Yes," stated the Lama. “Let me ask you a question. In a moment of physical ecstasy with your mate, have you ever screamed,'Oh, my God'?"

"I'm sure I have at one point or another, but..."

"But what?"

"I don't know that screaming out, 'Oh my God,' in a moment of ecstasy is going to give life to all things."

"Let me tell you," said the Lama, "that no life would exist without this vibration being present."

"You're telling me that the birds and the bees and everything in between is screaming, 'Oh my God,' so that their creation can happen?"

"When we want to create life, Jean, we go through what is known as the Five Elements of Creation. The First Element is the Divine Mind. This element holds the vision of the life we want to create. This vision is then lowered into the Second Element of Creation where this vision is filled with the Universal Life Force and given life through the sound of the vibration of the word, 'God.' This life force then enters into the Third Element of what is known as the soul where the memory of all our past lives is held. The soul then downloads our cellular memory into what is known as the Flower of Life that is held in the Fourth Element of the Etheric Plane or what you call Heaven. The Flower of Life projects onto the Fifth Element of the Physical Plane the sum total of who we are as humans. It is at this point that the doctor slaps our fanny in an effort to create enough energy to 'boot up' or turn on our brain and activate our hard drive or soul. Once complete then life begins as we know it here on earth."

"So you are saying that all life forms are created in this way?"

"Yes."

"You still haven't gotten around to explaining to me how you turned on the light inside you so we can see each other in this darkness."

"This light as you describe it is known as the Golden White Light of the Tao," the Lama said. "It is made up of the same seven colors at which each of us Lamas glow . When I say the word 'God' its vibration turns on all seven colors at once inside me and together do they glow in this white essence of light."

"For some reason I thought that you only glowed in one particular color."

"Each of the seven colors originate from what is known as the Universal Mind Substance. This is like the big computer in the sky. It continually uses each of the seven colors as a gateway into the physical body, much like you did in the entertainment business to transmit a proper reality free of stress and anxiety through the color red. Physical wellness is transmitted through the color orange. The color yellow enhances mental and physical performance. Physical and emotional pain are managed by the color green. Blue stimulates the longevity of life. The color indigo enhances the performance of the immune system to keep us free of disorder, and the color violet provides us with spiritual wellness."

"Well, if this is the case then why do we experience disorder?"

"Pain and suffering occur when stress is absorbed by the physical body. As this stress builds up, it begins to vibrate in jagged, eratic, up and down, pulses of energy. Over time this negative vibration becomes the dominant force in the body and invades these pure frequencies of light, changing them from a positive light force to a dark, stagnant energy that begins to break down the very essence of life."

"But isn't this the same idea that NASA was exploring when they introduced me to different frequencies that they believed the brain uses to run the software that manages our health?"

"In essence, yes. The difference," said the Lama, "is that for you or the astronauts to experience these frequencies depended on you all being connected to a brainwave machine."

"Yes, but..."

"Well, if all communication from the Universal Mind Substance (where all universal wisdom is held in perfection) is projected down to us on seven colors, it would have been easier for NASA to have individuals like yourself mentally project each color back to the astronauts with these vibrations of perfection, thus moving them out of whatever disorder they were experiencing."

"Oh my God, you are right. What an incredible idea." My mind had just jumped into hyper-drive.

"This is not an idea. This is how we communicate with you. We use these colors to travel from the Other Side to join you here on the physical plane."

"But I don't know if I would have the mental power needed to connect with the astronauts in space."

"What are you talking about?" said the Lama. “From the time His Holiness entered your body when you were four months old until now, you have been able to leave your physical body and cross over to the Other Side. "

"Excuse me! What are you talking about? His Holiness entering my body?"

"Yes, when you were four months old, His Holiness entered your body with the presence of his energy. Unfortunately, your little body had a hard time holding so much energy, and you began to convulse. Of course, it was these seizures that shot you out of your physical body to the Other Side where His Holiness met you so he could place his mark on you underneath your left arm."

"Hold it. My seizures were caused by my allergic reaction to my innoculations."

"I could see how the doctors would have come to that conclusion, but in fact, those seizures came about when His Holiness entered your body."

"But how about my autistic symptoms, my stuttering? They were very real to me."

"Oh, you did have those symptoms," said the Lama, “but they were the end result of having such a great amount of energy placed inside you by His Holiness."

"And, once again, why was I chosen to have such an experience?"

"You are always His Holiness’s voice when He appears every 26,000 years at the end of the earth's regenerational cycle."

AS A SIDE BAR

Right Now
Is All We Have Now
Right Now

Little did I know at the time, but the Lamas had manipulated my pain and suffering while in The Hole to force clarity on me so I could not only free myself of this pain and suffering but also help others along the way.

Clarity is seeing things as they actually are, and this is what we call wisdom. The voice of that wisdom is truth, and truth provides sincerity which gives integrity to all that we do. The majority of my time in isolation was spent in the meditation of clarity. Fortunately for me, I had spent the first two years of my life crossing over to the Other Side and over nine years doing research in a flotation tanks free of light, sound, and weight. I was able to reconstruct these memories while in the Hole and resolve all of my conflicts moment by moment. Once this karmic debt was removed, I was able to become the master of each moment. As each moment is experienced, I am able to see into that moment and take responsibility for its outcome. If the moment is taking more than giving, more negative than positive, then I say the word "God" and change the contents of this moment from a negative to a positive force that is working for me instead of against me as before.

Each second unfolds positively 86,400 times each day. Each day unfolds positively into the week then into the month. No longer is negative energy becoming karmic debt and stopping me from seeing reality as it actually is. My actual reality told me that being in jail was not a punishment. It was another Initiation created by the Lamas to test my ability to employ all that I had learned in such a way as to survive my ordeal without giving up my values or making a judgment.

The gods always give us two choices when deciding the right path to follow. One choice is seemingly the short cut to solving our problem. The other choice is seemingly the long way. The allure of the short cut is that our problem will be solved sooner than later as offered by the long way. Of course, by taking the short cut we have to give up some or all of our values, those things that determine our worth: integrity, fairness, respect for one another. The long way insures our values will stay intact, but to our way of thinking, will probably not provide a solution soon enough to meet our needs, especially if our needs are financial in nature. It would have been much easier for me to succumb to the government's wishes and turn over my clients. I would have been able to keep all of my possessions and circumvent the severe punishment acted out against me. This solution would have been the short cut. I would have failed my Initiation if I had taken this route. Judgment is very much a negative process. I was taught that any negative thought about another person was considered to be a judgment. I pondered this problem over and over in the quiet recesses of my mind. I thought about the actions of the G-Men toward me. My need to judge their actions against me made me their prisoner. Why? Because at the time I decide that someone or something was wrong in their actions. I had a conflict with them. The physical body becomes the karmic wheel ("like" energy attracting "like" energy) and draws me time and again to the person or situation with whom I have a conflict until I resolve it.

As we know, our ego forces us to set these conflicts aside instead of addressing them, thus continually putting us in front of those we least want to be in front of. In my situation, I wasn't able to sit down with the G-Men and resolve our conflict without giving up my values, but after many days of meditation, I reached a point of clarity and realized that there is a difference between judgment and observation. I can observe that someone is acting negatively towards me. At the point that I decide that they are wrong for acting this way, I have made a judgment, and once a judgment is made, a conflict arises. For their own particular reasons, the G-Men felt right in their actions against me. By freeing myself of the need to decide that they were wrong in their actions, I freed myself from being their prisoner. I unconditionally gave a gift of my energy to them. The G-Men then decided how they were going to use my gift. If they used my gift to take from me, I stepped back and gave them another unconditional gift of my energy, thus giving them another opportunity to use it properly. If they would have decided to return my gift to me in like kindness, then I would step forward and embrace them. If they chose, which they did more times than not, to take from me, then I stepped back once again, giving them an unconditional gift of my energy. This is called the Tai Chi of Events. Step forward, step back. Give and receive. After awhile of their taking and me giving, I built a force field of energy that protected me from their negative actions. This same energy force was then used by me to positively resolve my conflict with them but not before the G-Men had their last say.

FINAL PLAN...The G-Men Giveth and Taketh Away.

G Men
Government Force Right Of Course
No Recourse

During my time in jail, family members and friends were frantically searching for ways to get me out of jail before the G-Men decided that it might be easier to just get rid of me altogether. Finally, property that I owned outside the jurisdiction of my case was accepted as collateral for bail. A bail hearing was scheduled requiring my parents and those friends financially involved to travel to court and present evidence that said the property was not obtained through illegal means. This was not the kind of scenario that the G-Men wanted played out. Their fear was that once I was out on bail, I would tell my story and implicate all those involved. To stop this from happening, the G-Men made a visit one sunny morning to my lawyer's house and placed an illegal substance on the leather appointed front seat of his luxury car. When my lawyer entered the car, he sat on the illegal substance, and in doing so, sprang his own trap. The G-Men informed him of his rights and offered him the same deal that I had turned down. If he would inform on me, he would be set free. If, instead, he turned down their offer, then he would be sitting next to me in a hole of his own. My lawyer decided to take the short cut and keep his possessions while giving up his values, a small price to pay, or so he thought.

In the early morning I was dragged out of my hole and processed for release on bail. I was given the clothes that I had worn prior to my conversion to County Orange. Unfortunately, they no longer fit. Entering jail I weighed in at 185 lbs. Leaving county jail I weighed in at 132 lbs. I guess the Jew Balls did the trick. I was given an orientation on the many ways the government still owned me while out on bail and what my responsibilities would be once I was released. The only thing left for me to do was to turn the door knob and greet my loved ones on the other side. Wrong! The G-Men handcuffed me and began informing me of my rights. Evidently my bail had been revoked, and I would have to return to my hole. Why had my bail been revoked? My lawyer informed my parents and friends that my bail was to be revoked and there was no need to come to court. Since no one came to court, my bail was revoked. The G-Men thought that removing the opportunity to embrace my loved ones and returning me back to the hole would finally bring me around to their way of thinking. Their actions had the opposite affect on me. I was even more resolved to stand my ground and hold on to my values regardless of the consequences.

THE JUDGE LIKED BARBECUE

Judge Me
Not Today Just Let Me
Be Released

Two weeks after my near release, I was escorted back over to court to meet with the Assistant District Attorney assigned to my case. The meeting took place in a holding cell behind the court room. I had sat here numerous times before, watching a cross section of humanity crammed into this cell awaiting their fate. Due to the overcrowding, fights would break out. The deputies would be brought in to quell the event only to find out later that the culprit had, unfortunately, committed suicide. My fate would be less severe. The Assistant District Attorney offered me the opportunity to give him the information requested or spend the next 18 months in jail. I refused to accommodate their offer while my attorney pleaded with me to give them what they wanted. I immediately found myself in front of the judge for final sentencing.

I was barely able to stand upright before the judge. My weakened condition and the presence of light conjured up a likeness of Howard Hughes in his final days.

The judge spoke. "I understand by looking over your records that you grew up close to me. Are you familiar with my parent's restaurant, the Bar B Q Corral?"

All I could do to respond was to shake my head up and down in an action of affirmation.

"Well, this is your lucky day," said the judge. "Looking over your records, it seems as though the government has had their way with you for quite some time. They have stomped all over your civil rights and threatened you with bodily harm if you failed to succumb to their demands. I am ordering a complete review of this case and all that is involved. I am giving you probation. You are free to leave."

It sounded like a wooden shoe convention when all the jaws dropped to the floor. Everyone was jumping up and down and yelling at the judge saying how unfair his judgment was. I, instead, collapsed and fell to the floor.

My next recollection was going through the same release process, only to find that this time I did walk through the door out into a very bright and blinding world. I couldn't see. I stumbled and fell back against the door. My eyes burned. I couldn't focus. I became disoriented. Suddenly I was grabbed by the arm and jerked around. Although I couldn't see my assailant, I recognize the voice of the G-Man.

"Don't think we're finished with you. You are still our property," said the G-Man.

The Lamas were right. I had better change my name before the G-Men killed me.

ARE YOU REAL?

A Dream?
Are You Real Are You
There Where?

All of a sudden I realized that someone was trying to help me back to my feet. I turned to see what I thought was an illusion in the form of my fiance', Colleen.

"Colleen." I whispered.

"Oh my God!... Jean, what have they done to you?" Unbeknownst to Colleen, it was me she was helping to my feet. She thought she was just helping this degenerate of a figure with long, straggly hair, wearing clothes twice as big as his frame, unable to see and too weak to stand.

My next memory was waking up in bed with Colleen lying next to me. This had to be a dream. I pinched myself and let out a sound of pain which woke up Colleen. Still unconvinced, I pinched Colleen, and she flinched and recoiled back into the pillow.

"What did you do that for?" she said.

"I wanted to know if you are real."

CHAPTER SEVEN

Back Home
Not For Long Wrong Again
No Win

BACK TO TAOS, NEW MEXICO

I returned to Taos, New Mexico in the summer of '86 to knock the cobwebs away from the door and reopen my research facility. So many things had happened since its conception: mind/body exploration, sensory deprivation research, cranial electrical restructuring, development of performance training while rockin 'n' rollin, the dolphins and my initiation through incarceration. It all left me in a quandary as to where to begin. The Lamas had already decided where I should start. They thought I should learn how to join my spiritual and physical bodies together as One. As always they went about it in the most unusual way.

GOOD NEWS! BAD NEWS!

Grand Jury
Wielding Power From a Tower
Justice Sours

In August of '86, I received word from the court that employed the infamous G-Men that they were going to rewrite history and free me of the charges that had tested my values and integrity and threatened their sense of safety in their own penal system. The only problem was that I had to return and appear in front of those same judges that had called this circus to order in the first place.

Upon arriving at the courthouse steps, I was greeted by my lawyer.

"Well, I have some good news and some bad news."

"Tell me the good news," I said.

"Well, you don't have to go back to jail."

"What do you mean I don't have to go back to jail? I thought I was being being released from my charges."

Grand Jury
So Regal Bend Ya Over
Legal Eagle

"The powers that be have decided to enact another grand jury investigation in your honor, and if you are willing to tell them what you know, then they will drop all charges. If not, then you're going back to jail."

Once again, I refused their request and went back to jail.

For some reason the G-Men thought that once I got settled back into my lifestyle, I would feel more of a need to cooperate, especially if it was going to be taken away from me again. WRONG!!!

What the G-Men did not understand was that I did not consider this to be a punishment as much as another Initiation by the Lamas. As long as I held fast to my values and integrity, I would always come out on top.

ONCE AGAIN..BACK IN TAOS.. THIS TIME IN FRONT OF MASTER E CHU

E Chu
Tai Chi Master Powerful Force
His Way

I had been back in Taos from my extended stay with the G-Men for just about a month when I found myself standing in line at the post office to receive whatever mail had been sent my way. This particular morning was like most others except for the fact that my attention was drawn to a small Chinese man standing off to the side trying to fill out a Return Receipt Requested Form, something that I knew quite a bit about, since most legal responses as related to land transactions are sent in this manner. I took the opportunity to present myself to this person and offer assistance.

"Maybe I can be of help."

"Thank you so much," said the man. "Forms confusing."

"No problem," I said. "Are you visiting?"

"Here to find person," he said in broken English

.

"Who might that person be? I may know the person you're looking for."

"I'm looking for man whose name Jean Genet. Would you know this man?"

You could hear my chin crash to the floor as I struggled to regain my composure.

"I'm Jean Genet! Why are you looking for me?"

"The Lamas send me. I teach you Tai Chi."

"Tai Chi?" I asked with a somewhat puzzled look on my face.

"Tai Chi is where, through breathing and physical movement, you join spiritual-physical bodies together as One...create a force strong enough to radiate out from you and touch right people and events that bring about right opportunities to create great abundance for you."

Over the next year Master E Chu and I practiced the graceful movements of Tai Chi to join our physical and spiritual bodies together as One so we can always be at the right place and time to be of service and receive our abundance. We crossed over to the Other Side to meet with the Lamas and learn Astral Projection Meditation so we can provide "remote healing" to the world. I became the Master of the Now where all attachments to people and events are released and we embrace each other in the happiness of the moment.

On one particular night, Master E Chu and I were sitting inside my research center. Candles were lighting the interiors, creating a meditative state, when a strong vibrational presence made itself known. One of the Lamas decided to join us.

"Master E Chu. How are you?" The Lama had a nice, warm, tone in his voice.

"Too much time since last visit," Master E Chu welcomed the Lama.

"So how is our student doing in his training?" the Lama asked.

"Slowly but surely things in his life beginning to come full circle and complete themselves. No longer indecisive. His focus becoming sharp. His intentions strong. He becoming master of his moment. If the moment negative, he takes responsibility to change energy to positive force."

The Lama directed his attention toward me.

"Jean, where do you find yourself at in this process?"

"Before I had always tried to control the future by setting goals, getting an education, securing the right job with the right mate in the right home at the right time to have children, and having enough life insurance to protect us against what we couldn't control. Now I take charge of each moment and insure that the moment becomes positive. Each positive moment flows into each hour that makes up the totality of my day and becomes my future, a future filled with all the positive moments of my existence, filled now with abundance."

"Master E Chu, I believe you have something to give Jean," the Lama said.

With that, Master E Chu reached in back of him and brought forth a package that was wrapped in the same type of paper with which the Mandala had been covered.

"Here, Jean Genet," Master E Chu said. "This you have earned."

I began to unfold the paper carefully, when Master E Chu interrupted.

"Tear it. Nothing special," as Master E Chu reached over and tore the package open.

Inside was a beautiful ceremonial robe.

"My master's robe," said Master E Chu. "Now yours."

I was dumbfounded. I sat there looking at this ancient robe.

"Go ahead. Try it on," said the Lama.

I got to my feet, reached down and grasped the robe with my fingers and brought the robe up to my shoulders. I was being unsuccessful in getting my arms into the sleeves of the robe due to the fact that each arm hole contained such a large opening.

"Student," Master E Chu grunted as he popped up and held the backside of the robe straight across so I could insert my arms.

As I wrapped the robe around me, I immediately felt a

surge of energy engulf me from inside the robe. It was as if a force field of energy had surrounded me.

"You now Master" said Master E Chu.

With that response the Lama and Master E Chu both began to vibrate. Their individual "light" merged into one and exited out the open window.

My training with Master E Chu had come to a close.

The Lamas had been successful in bringing my spiritual and physical bodies together as one whole being. With new vision I decided to bring all of my research full circle. Two years elapsed in what seemed to be the wink of an eye, but in that time I determined what methods of self exploration brought about the best results in the shortest period of time.

Once the bridge was successfully crossed between the mind and the body, the opportunities were endless for its use. I could dominate any field that could benefit from having mental clarity, physical vitality, emotional balance, and financial abundance that supports spiritual wellness. But what field would most benefit? That was the question. The answer came from an unlikely source, *Rolling Stone* magazine.

NO SOLUTIONS..."I FEEL LIKE I'VE BEEN ROLLED OVER BY A STONE."

Chronic Fatigue
Tired Disorder Before Your Time
Runs Out

In my quandry to find a suitable market for my wares, I came across an article in *Rolling Stone* magazine about Epstein-Barr Virus or Yuppie Disease. The author was a lady who was suffering from this mysterious disorder that created extreme fatigue while creating havoc in her mental, physical, and emotional body. She felt that there were no solutions to address her condition.

As I read the article (There are no accidents.), I began to realize that while out on tour, entertainers and their support personnel suffered from similar symptoms that I called "fatigue that was chronic." I drafted a letter to *Rolling Stone* detailing my experience with this type of fatigue while out on tour, explaining that I didn't think it was a virus as much as it was stress entering the body and distorting the brain's ability to enter into the proper frequencies for regeneration. The solution was to properly realign the brain's frequencies, and in doing so, move out of the reality of fatigue into a reality of wellness.

My letter was passed on to the National Epstein-Barr Virus Foundation, and they in turn invited me to speak with their largest support group in Denver, Colorado. Eventually, my views were passed along with those of many others to the Center For Disease Control in Atlanta, Georgia, and out of this came the term, "Chronic Fatigue," a term that was too soft for such a debilitating disorder. Eventually, I would begin to call this disorder Aging Genetic Elevator or A.G.E.

GEORGE WASHINGTON WOULD BE PROUD

Cherry Trees
Cut Down Replanted Start Over
New Home

I saw a great opportunity to create a new research model that would develop the technology necessary to move the brain back into the reality of wellness, free of fatigue, and explore this new demon, Chronic Fatigue. In turn, it would provide me with a sufficient number of clients whom I could put into the water with dolphins and see if their health improved from the experience.

I decided to stay in Denver and look for a suitable facility that would give me the opportunity to design this new research model, but first I needed a mailing address.

As always, the most amazing things happen when you realize that there are no accidents, and the karmic tumblers landed on three god's eyes across the board.

There is a post office in a section of Denver called Cherry Creek. The city fathers have seen fit over the years to cut down most of the cherry trees that gave the area its name (George Washington would be proud.) to give way to development that required the builders to plant new cherry trees.

Walking along the sidewalk on my way to get a post office box, I was stopped by a voice that said, "Where are you going?" I turned to see a red headed leprechaun of a man sitting on a bench in front of storefront underneath a sign that read, "Post Haste."

"I'm going to rent a post office box," I said hesitantly.

"Well, this is your lucky day," said Freddy. "I have such a box for rent here in my store."

Post Haste was owned by Freddy Rudlet, a retired hospital administrator. Freddy was the first to establish Flight for Life helicopter rescue. He introduced massage therapy and acupuncture into a hospital setting. Freddy was in the forefront of joining the mind into the body for all around healing at a time when the medical profession associated such behavior with witch doctors.

After retirement Freddy decided to address another problem in society ... the Post Office. Long lines drove Freddy right up the wall, so he solved the problem by opening up his own Post Haste next door to the Post Office.

I immediately made friends with Freddy and leased a box in the name of the North Star Trust. My father always told me if I ever got lost to just look up into the sky, find the North Star, and trust that it would lead me home. Well, I felt at home in Denver.

Within a short period of time, I began to receive mail under the name of Nustar. I confronted Freddy with the problem.

"Oh, you evidently need to meet Steve Stevens."

"Why do I need to meet this man Stevens?" I asked.

"He is developing a brain wave machine of some sorts."

The Lamas had rolled the karmic tumblers once again. There are no accidents.

Steve Stevens had been a research assistant for a man by the name of Michael Hercules who had originally led the team that developed the Brain Entrainment Technology or CES / Cranial Electrical Stimulus for which NASA employed me out of Vietnam as a consultant and which the astronauts used while in space to address their mental and emotional stress as it related to their physical performance. It is also the area of research that I had funded through the National Center For Integrative Medicine.

I set an appointment with Steve to meet at my apartment and exchange the mail.

Each time I move to another home, I immediately set up my flotation tank and my computer. When Steve arrived he entered into an efficiency apartment furnished with one futon or sleeping mat, the flotation tank, and the computer. The Lamas would be impressed with the simplicity.

I was impressed with what Steve brought with him. It was a prototype of a Brain Entrainment Device / BED that was about the size of a paperback book. With new microcircuitry Steve had created in miniature form a Brain Entrainment Device that an individual could take home. Before it would have been impossible due to the fact that the old BED machines were large and cumbersome, requiring the patient to come to the device. Steve and I immediately joined forces to integrate our research so we could fine tune the mind and put the body in the proper reality of wellness, thus freeing it of Chronic Fatigue.

THE NATIONAL RESEARCH CENTER FOR CHRONIC FATIGUE WAS BORN

Unlikely Spot
Float Home to Cure Fatigue
Ready Go

Steve and I had our own separate tools to begin the process of research and development. The problem was that these tools needed to be housed under the same roof.

Once again, while reading the newspaper, I came across an advertisement for the sale of a flotation tank. I called the number provided and found out that the tank was stored in the back of what had been, at one time, a private steam room for men. I made an appointment to see the tank and was given an address, but when I arrived I was surprised to find out that the old steam room had been converted into a ten thousand square foot medical clinic. I was led past the newest in chiropractic, acupuncture, and massage therapy with a huge sauna and whirlpool to an area in the very back that housed the tank. It was apparent that the tank had not been used in quite some time. Salt was encrusted from the inside out with little chance that it could be used in its present condition.

I began to ask several tank related questions only to find out that the person I really needed to talk to would be available shortly. Just then a man came through the door, extended his hand, and said, "Hi, I'm Brian Martin. So you want to buy this salt tank?"

"I don't know. I already have one tank," I said, "and to fix this one up and move it to my apartment would leave me no room to do anything but float around."

"Well, move your tank over here. That would solve the problem."

The National Research Center for Chronic Fatigue had found a home.

Norm and Barb.
all the best,
Jean

CHAPTER EIGHT

Computer Chip
Will Make You Sick So
Don't Eat

CHIPPING AWAY AT OUR HEALTH

When I was growing up in the 50's, there was little sign of stress-related disorders. There was the occasional child who always seemed to be stricken with Leukemia. The elderly were experiencing loss of memory on their way out of their body into the next life. Polio had been conquered. T.B. seemed to be a thing of the past.

What caused a shift to occur that moved us away from relatively good health and started what we now consider to be an epidemic with stress related disorders? As a researcher you look for the one thing that presents itself, and with its presence, starts this negative shift toward ill health in our society.

I believe the shift occurred with the introduction back in the early 60's of the computer chip. Everything is now run with some sort of computer chip. I would be hard pressed to find much in our society that does not have the presence of a computer chip somewhere in its makeup.

So what is the big deal about the presence of computer chips in our society, and how can something so small have such a negative effect on our health?

As I have mentioned before, I believe that during our sleep cycle the brain repairs us mentally, physically, emotionally, and spiritually by moving us out of the reality of our discomfort into a reality that is free of whatever is bothering us, thus repairing or healing us. When we first begin to nod out and move away from a conscious, awakened state into the subconscious or sleep state, the brain, in an effort to gain enough energy to completely repair or heal us, moves us out of the reality of stress and anxiety through a door into a reality that is free of stress and anxiety. The brain does this by creating a frequency that my philosophy of Tje Jan believes is received from the energy of the sun, the moon, and the twenty-eight constellations. We only see this energy after a rain when the sun shines through the rain drops and reflects the seven colors of the rainbow: violet, indigo, blue, green, yellow, orange, and red. Each one of these colors creates a specific frequency that our brain receives and uses to unlock this door so we can move through it and find our way to the Other Side or what I would call the spiritual body. We absorb this healing energy in our spiritual body long enough to heal or repair us, then the doorway opens once again and returns us to our physical body free of stress and anxiety. There is a specific frequency for physical healing. A certain frequency also unlocks the door to our mental and emotional well being. There's a doorway into super learning as there is a doorway into cellular regeneration and spiritual well being.

When stress enters the body from whatever source, be it the energy that comes off our television/entertainment centers, radar oven, an alarm clock too close to our head, our refrigerator, lighting systems, our automobile's computers, electric blankets or overhead power lines, its structure becomes twisted, spiraling in its movement. As it spirals inside us, stress creates a vibration that emits a frequency of its own. Once integrated with the healing frequencies of the brain, it changes the dynamics or structure of these frequencies and opens doors into realities that hold the environment of stress-related disorders. The more the stress, the more the dynamics of the healing frequency change, the more severe the symptoms of the disorder seem to become.

What is the one thing that seems to distort or change the healing frequencies of the brain the most? That's right. It's the energy of the computer chip.

GETTING OLD WHILE WE'RE YOUNG

I'm Young
Why Do I Feel Old
Can't Remember

Over our lifetimes our bodies move through different stages of health. It seems the older we get, the less energy we have to be proficient in our mental, emotional, and physical skills. These stages are more acceptable the older we get. If we are in our 80's we accept the fact that we will mentally begin to forget the small things, hoping to remember the large ones. We accept our physical limitations and become more emotionally detached from the realities of age until we complete the process of separating from our physical body so that our spiritual being can cross over to the other side or heaven. What we cannot accept is being mentally, physically, and emotionally challenged long before our time, especially if these challenges manifest into a stress-related disorder that takes away our life force, eventually ending our existence as we know it. This is why I believe, as I mentioned before, the term Chronic Fatigue does not adequately describe the seriousness of this disorder.

Anything that accelerates the life process to such an extent that you begin to experience the final stages of your life while you are still young should be called Aging Genetic Elevator or A.G.E.

When Chronic Fatigue/A.G.E. was first recognized back in the mid 80's as an ailment, the age span affected seemed to be between the late 30's and the mid 60's and was most recognizable in women with professional careers. Within one year the disorder expanded to include not only professionals but children as young as six. The common thread among the children afflicted with A.G.E. was their interest and extensive use of entertainment devices (cassette players/CD's with headphones, TV's), a variety of appliances, and, of course, computers. Another factor that was common to this stress-related scenario was the professions of the parents. The higher the stress of the parents' profession, the more it seemed to manifest onto the child. The relationship of the parents to one another played a very important role in determining the extent of the stress felt by the child, especially if the child's personality caused him or her to feel the need to mediate between the different factions of the family. In these cases the more severe disorders a child experienced, the closer the home seemed to be to overhead power lines.

I don't know anyone in today's society who doesn't show the symptoms of A.G.E. Do you know anyone who does not have occasional headaches, sleepless nights, loss of memory (however slight), tiredness, and frequent emotional outbursts? These symptoms are now so common in our society that we accept them as a natural part of our stress-related environment. Oh, we may combat A.G.E. by having stress management courses. Management is the key word. We don't do anything to get rid of the stress. We only have time to manage it.

A portion of our A.G.E. clients were individuals who did what one would think to be the right action, work out. I had clients who ran several miles a day, lifted weights, and did aerobics. Unfortunately, stress is not reduced by working out. If anything, working out only accelerates fatigue. What actually happens is that the person who works out to reduce stress is too tired at the end of the workout to feel the fatigue.

We now move on to explore how our sleep cycle determines the condition of our health.

THE SLEEP CYCLE IS THE INTERNET TO OUR HEALTH

Can't Sleep
Wake Up Tired I Ache
Well "Da"

Remember when I mentioned that the brain is a computer, and that the functions of the body, seeing, tasting, hearing, smelling, speaking, movement, etc., are software programs that the brain/computer manages? The brain, just like a computer, needs energy to run these programs. When stress moves the brain into negative realities that take energy, the brain begins to lose the ability to manage these programs properly.

In our sleep cycle, the brain moves from our conscious being into what is known as the Alpha state. At this level, the brain moves into a reality that is free of stress and anxiety, and it is in this reality that we absorb enough energy to physically heal ourselves.

The brain then moves into the Theta state of awareness where we enter into environments that enhance our performance mentally, physically, and emotionally. Theta is also the level of awareness where the left side of the brain, which operates off a particular frequency, conceptualizes or mentally thinks about what the physical body is to do and how the physical body will emotionally feel about what it is doing. The left side joins with the right side of the brain which operates on a different frequency, causing it to act on the directions the left side of the brain has given it. This harmonic state (joining more than one frequency together, in this case, the left and right sides of the brain) is known as the meditative state of awareness. It is here where we enter through a door that moves us out of our physical body into our spiritual state of being. It is in this spiritual state, free of the demands of the physical body, that the brain absorbs enough energy to physically heal our body.

The brain then moves deeper into the Theta state of awareness where we now enter into environments that enhance our performance mentally, physically, and emotionally. I believe that it is in this spiritual state, free of the demands of the physical body, that the brain no longer releases enough of the experiences of our day through the process of dreaming that the brain does not have enough energy to recall those things that it has decided to keep in its memory. When we are old this inability to remember is called senility. When we are experiencing A.G.E. we call it Alzheimers.

It has been my experience that a person stricken with Alzheimers is not experiencing the deterioration of the brain as much as s/he is unable to move through the proper door to access the reality that holds his/her memory. Once the person accesses the frequency that opens up the door to his/her memory, then the act of remembering is easier. As our brain releases more and more of the memories of the day and regains energy while in the Theta state, the brain seems to use this energy to address chronic emotional and physical pain. Once the brain completes its dream cycle and regains enough energy to open up the proper doors, then the physical and emotional bodies are moved through these doors into the proper realities for repair/healing. Another benefit of hanging out in the Theta state is the ability to absorb wisdom.

Once the path is clear of mental, physical, and emotional blocks, the individual is free to stand once again in the light of what the Lamas call the Universal Mind Substance. It is in this state of awareness that we experience the sum total of all the spiritual realities. This golden light is the energy of the Universal Mind Substance shining all the wisdom of the universe onto our being. We absorb this wisdom into our cells and store it in our soul so we can intuitively live out this wisdom in our service to others.

What a magnificent process!

The final stage of our sleep cycle is known as the Delta state of awareness. Here doorways are available to promote the longevity of life processes and provide spiritual healing. Aging Genetic Elevator (A.G.E.) raises its ugly head as stress enters the body and once again changes the frequencies the brain uses to open up the right doors into the proper realities of health.

As I mentioned before, the brain warns us much like the warning light on the dashboard of our car. We have a tendency to pay more attention to the warning light on the dashboard than we do to the subtle signals our brain uses when it creates tiredness, headaches, sleepless nights, depression, and loss of memory. Once again, we feel that the headaches, the fatigue, the depression, are part of living in our hectic environment. At some point when the brain has lost a sufficient amount of energy by absorbing too much stress, A.G.E. is triggered, and the brain loses more of its ability to enter and maintain the Delta state of awareness. At that point people begin to lose the spiritual balance and sense of who they are. They question their relationship to themselves, family, friends, and their job. They become spiritually lost.

As stress builds up and further drains the brain's battery, it loses more of its ability to manage the cellular processes that relate to the immune system, allowing more colds with flu-like symptoms. The mental and physical processes that the Theta state of awareness manages begin to wane and the person shows signs of fatigue such as going to bed tired, waking up tired, inability to form complete thoughts, loss of attention, the start of headaches, some memory loss, depression, and the beginning of nightmares. As negative as depression and on-going physical and mental fatigue seem to be, the brain uses them as tools to slow the person down in an effort to conserve energy.

Once again, these are all warning signs the brain is using in an effort to get our attention and move us into action. If no action is taken, then our brain has a harder time maintaining and enhancing not only our mental and emotional performance but also the physical processes that the Alpha state of awareness manages. This is very evident with sports figures who go into the proverbial slump. This slump becomes habitual with A.G.E. and unfortunately, as we were to find out, we also create a habit of being sick.

THE HABIT OF BEING SICK

It Seems
Like I'm Always Sick Habit
I Guess

As part of its memory process, our brain recognizes every environment in which we function and survive. When the sports figure strikes out at the plate, the brain memorizes the time of day, the temperature, the color of the sky, the smell of resin, the view of the fans, the players on the field, and the sense of the catcher and umpire standing behind him. All of these things are recorded by the brain, so when the player steps up to the plate again, the brain views the current environment, matches it to what it has experienced before, and plays back the same memory, and within that memory the batter strikes out. The brain, being a computer, doesn't know that it is wrong to strike out; the brain only knows that the batter survived under thc same environmental conditions. Each time the same batter steps up to the plate in the same game under the same conditions, he has an 80% chance of striking out again.

This same process occurs when stress moves the brain into the negative environment of A.G.E. The brain memorizes where we are when the symptoms of depression, headaches, mental, and physical fatigue occur. When we move back into that environment, whether it be our house, our automobile, work, or anywhere we travel, the brain matches the current environment with what it has in its memory and recreates our response to the environment, which includes reenacting our symptoms. Remember, the brain only gives us back what we put into it. The brain does not know that having the symptoms of A.G.E. is bad. The brain only knows that we survived last time we were in the same environment. It is this process of recreating the same negative effects time and time again that causes mental, physical, and emotional pain to become chronic or A.G.E. The less the brain is able to enter into its dream cycle to release these negative memories that have now become habitual, the more this negative energy distorts the brain's ability to manage the body and the more severe the symptoms of A.G.E. become until such a time that the symptoms become part of the brain's permanent memory and begin to display themselves as ailments. An ailment is many symptoms put together to form a picture of how the disorder will affect us mentally, physically, or emotionally. The genetic profile of the individual will determine (1) where the ailment will affect us, in the lungs, heart, stomach, kidney, etc., and (2) when the ailment manifests as a disorder. In my family, my mother's side of the family is more prone to diabetes, where my father's side is more prone to heart disease.

The severity of the ailments displayed will determine what stage of A.G.E we are experiencing. I believe there are five stages of A.G.E.. The stages of A.G.E. are provided on the following pages.

THE FIVE STAGES OF A.G.E.

Stage One

- Going to bed tired.
- Sleeping disorders, tossing and turning, waking up at irregular hours.
- Waking up tired.
- Muscle aches.
- Depression.
- Confused thinking, inability to see the beginning, the middle or the end of problems, personal or business.
- Small memory loss: names, telephone numbers, recent/ current events.
- Headaches, mild to moderate, usually lasting an hour or so.
- Nervous stomach, reaction to spicy foods, mild indigestion, heartburn.

Stage Two

- Sleeping disorders now become defined.
- Restlessness becomes more pronounced.
- The person cannot settle into sleeping postures, sleeps very lightly, and is easily awakened.
- Nightmares start. Tiredness is prolonged.
- Muscle aches are becoming more noticeable.
- Some swelling of joints develops.
- Depression turns to anxiety.
- Feeling of emptiness manifests.
- Problems are no longer defined separately, i.e., work, mate, family.
- Life is now a problem.

- Memory loss becomes more pronounced.
- Past events in one's life lose form.
- Headaches now become more frequent, more severe. Headache is now constant for most of the day, tolerable but painful.
- Stomach's reaction to general food groups, including spicy foods, becomes more severe. Indigestion becomes more prevalent, longer lasting. Heartburn intensifies, especially in early morning hours. Low grade fevers begin to occur.
- The person is more susceptible to colds that turn into prolonged bouts with the flu.
- Immune system begins to weaken.

Stage Three

- Sleeping provides no relief.
- The person becomes afraid to go to sleep.
- Nightmares now become horrific.
- Individual wakes up void of feeling.
- Tiredness is now classified as "bone tired."
- Mental, physical, and emotional exhaustion is now constant.
- Muscle and joint soreness and swelling now become severe.
- Symptoms point toward arthritis, lupus.
- Headaches are classified as "migraine."
- Nausea, blurred vision can occur separately or together.
- The severity of the pain might increase to a nagging headache. The length of the headache is now measured in days instead of hours.
- Depression has now become severe. The emptiness of feeling now provokes thoughts of possible suicide.

- Person feels all solutions to problems exhausted.
- Anxiety is now producing emotional imbalance and quickness to erupt over the slightest provocation.
- Emotional fear has now set in.
- Memory loss is severe, showing same symptoms as Alzheimers Disease. For example, in a department store, a person walks down the pot and pan aisle, picks up a tea pot, but the mind is blank as to its identity or use. The person looks down the aisle, cannot identify the purpose of the aisle, cannot remember what store he is in, or why he came. Anxiety begins to set in, and he loses complete recollection of location, store, city, home, state, etc. He begins to feel claustrophobic.
- Stomach disorders now showing symptoms of ulcers with severe burning abdominal pain.
- Organs (kidneys, lungs, liver, heart) show signs of dysfunction.
- Cellular imbalance.
- Symptoms related to possible cancer, lupus, arthritis, etc.
- Lack of balance control while standing.

Stage Four

- Debilitating disorder has now moved from an ailment to an affliction.

Stage Five

- Death

The value of having the five stages of A.G.E. to refer to is obvious. We can match those A.G.E. symptoms that move the brain's frequencies back into alignment so the proper reality can be accessed for repair. The reality of the results went way beyond our expectations. We can match the symptoms the patient is experiencing with the stage that provides a clearer picture of his particular makeup. With this information in hand, we can determine which frequencies the brain is not accessing and use the Brain Entrainment Device to move the brain's frequencies back into alignment so the proper reality can be accessed for repair. The reality of the results went way beyond our expectations.

A NUSTAR ON THE HORIZON

A Device
To Release The Vice On
The Brain

During the time we were exploring the in's and out's of A.G.E., Steve Stevens was putting the final touches on his Brain Entrainment Device. In any form of development, it seems to be an endless process of design and application. You try one thing and it works up to a point, then it triggers an unwanted response. Then you adjust for that response only to find out that the adjustment just brought about another reaction that was undesirable to the overall function of the device. Sound confusing? Well, it is even more so when you are trying to have different frequencies integrate properly into an overall response from a device that is no larger than a small paper back book. Our up front work in defining the stages of A.G.E. helped determine which frequencies would best unlock the doors into those realities that repair us mentally, physically, emotionally, and spiritually. Choosing the correct frequency was a fairly simple process once we found a way to measure the subject's response to the frequency itself.

At the time, the general consensus of the medical community was that any response from the patient on how he was experiencing the condition of his health, good, bad or ugly, was invalid due to the fact that the patient had no medical education on which to base a correct decision. I thought that the patient's response was the most valuable, since the patient was doing the experiencing.

We decided to create a "before and after" response form. We wanted to measure to what extent the patient was feeling stress, and how stress affected the patient's mental, physical, emotional, and spiritual being. We provided a definition of stress, a feeling of being agitated, on edge, tense. We would then ask the subject to rate how they were experiencing this stress with "ten" being the worst, "zero" being completely free of stress, and "five" describing a mean average of how they usually felt when stress was present. We would then put the subject on the Brain Entrainment Device at the particular frequency we felt would best move the subject out of the reality of stress into one free of stress and anxiety.

After the session was over, we would solicit the subject's response and take note of the difference. For example, if before the session started the subject felt he was experiencing stress at the level of "eight," with "ten" being the worst, and then measured a "four" after the session, then the patient reduced his stress by 50%. The subject now had a simple way of measuring his or her repair or healing. The brain also recognizes this difference and begins to create a habit of healing. This form of measurement is known as META Analysis.

With this information in hand, we were able to decide exactly which frequencies provided the best response for repair of the mental, physical, emotional, and spiritual bodies. Steve then included these frequencies into what he called the Nustar, a Brain Entrainment Device that would open up the proper doorways for us to travel to new horizons of well being and freedom from the symptoms of A.G.E.. To bring the process full circle, we now needed to embrace the energy of the dolphins and begin to repair the spiritual body of the soul.

CHAPTER NINE

We Humans
Evolved From Dolphins You Sea
Me Flipper

THE DOLPHINS FLIPPED A.G.E. UPSIDE DOWN

I arrived in the Florida Keys. The Keys are a grouping of some twenty-nine coral islands south of Miami.

Legend has pirates forcing the Spanish galleons into the reefs and relieving them of their treasures. This jungle-like environment is lush with tropical flowers, coral-filled blue waters, summer temperatures that squeeze the mercury readings into the top of the thermometer with the humidity forcing salty liquid from the pores of your skin like a myriad of waterfalls. Arriving from the cool rocky mountain waters that fill up Coors beer cans, I couldn't have moved into a harsher environment, but for the dolphins it was most desirable.

I immediately began to research dolphins. Dolphins have been around some 45 million years. In our present form, we have been around some 50,000 years. We have the same skeletal and organ structure as the dolphin. We have a similar cerebral form. Our finger configurations are like what the dolphins have in their pectoral fins. In the first nine months of our gestation, the human fetus is much like a dolphin. The dolphin has three more months to configure their rostrum or extended jaw bone, develop their dorsal and pectoral fins, and finally, their fluke or tail section, all of which identifies them as a dolphin.

In other words, there is mounting evidence that suggests that our common ancestors might be dolphins.

What is even more important to understand about dolphins is that they are voluntary breathers. In other words, they have to think about taking a breath. Dolphins cannot sleep due to the fact that they wouldn't be able to consciously know when to take a breath. To regenerate, the dolphins have a brain that is "double wired." One brain turns OFF to charge its batteries while the other side switches ON, and not only manages all the functions of its body, but does it in such a way as to provide mental clarity, physical vitality, and emotional balance to the dolphin. If my assumption is that dolphins are our common ancestors, then there is the possibility that humans also have access to these same qualities.

I believe I have located where these "switches" are in humans, and most important, I believe I know how to turn these Switches ON.

To prove this I invited those suffering from A.G.E. to join me in the Florida Keys. This tropical island atmosphere offered a release from the environment in which these A.G.E. sufferers had been living. Just to have the warmth of the sun on their faces and the blue color of the sky reflecting in their eyes moved them into a much needed sense of peace and quiet.

Then stepping into the warm waters of the Atlantic Ocean

and feeling the presence of the dolphins around them seem to give them the added strength necessary to begin the process of embracing a new life free of A.G.E..

Before entering the water with the dolphins, blood was drawn from each subject to create a DNA profile. Every disorder that effects the physical makeup of the human body is displayed in the DNA as a separate code or what is called a "marker." Once this marker was located, we had a brain map done to determine the level of conscious awareness and then turned ON the switches.

After the swim concluded, the person was subjected to another brain mapping to get a sense of what s/he was experiencing on a mental, physical, and emotional level. After each dolphin encounter, the swimmer reported a sense of inner calmness while experiencing an outward feeling of exhilaration. The brain map confirmed that the dolphins had indeed moved the swimmer into the high end of the Alpha state. This is the area of the subconscious that opens the door and moves us into a reality free of stress and anxiety.

This was a very important find. Before this discovery we could only access the healing effects of the subconscious when we were asleep. Now with the help of the dolphins, we could begin to access the healing centers of the subconscious while awake.

In the prior swim sessions, the dolphins could only move the participant into the upper levels of the Alpha state. Although the release of stress and anxiety contributed greatly to the overall feelings of wellness within each individual, we needed to access the other levels of repair the subconscious had to offer.

In the next series of swims, we turned on their switches and used the Nustar to first move the swimmer into the reality that was free of physical pain. In the next swim the participant experienced the environment that enhanced performance. Another session opened the doorway so memory could be accessed. Before the next dolphin encounter, the swimmer moved into the reality free of fatigue. The swimmer then mentally participated in the reality of enhanced performance of their immune system. In the final session the participant crossed over into a spiritual reality of wholeness. Brain mapping confirmed the ability of the dolphins to use their echolocation to access the frequency the Nustar had created within the subconscious of the swimmer and to expand its dynamics to accelerate the response of repair and healing on all mental, physical, emotional, and spiritual planes.

As I mentioned earlier, we believe that when you first enter into the water with the dolphins, the dolphins sound you with their echolocation. This energy comes from the forehead of the dolphin in the form of clicking sounds at such a high vibration that it literally integrates with the etheric body of energy around the physical structure of the swimmer. This information is then returned to the dolphin, transforming the dolphin into the mental, physical, emotional, and spiritual pattern of the swimmer. If the swimmer is mentally disturbed, the dolphin becomes mentally disturbed. If the swimmer is emotionally upset, the dolphin becomes emotionally upset. If the swimmer is experiencing physical pain, the dolphin will feel the physical pain in the same area as the swimmer. Every square inch of the dolphin's surface is sensitized to receive and feel information from its surroundings including the physical pain emitting from the swimmer. To bring this information into spiritual balance, the dolphin changes the vibration of its brainwaves and moves through those doors whose environment on the Other Side is free of the negative aspects of the swimmer's environment. This exchange between the dolphin and the human through "thought transference" is experienced while floating in an ocean of salt water. Salt water is trillions of liquid crystals reflecting the new reality of the dolphin back onto the swimmer free of all the negative elements of the gross physical body.

We now know that although the frequencies dolphins use are very similar to our own, they differ in that these dolphins' frequencies are made up of more harmonics. Frequencies provide a much deeper experience when there are more layers or harmonics inside them. This was proven when we did another DNA profile on our swimmers only to find out that the marker that before had identified the presence of the disorder had completely dissolved, thus proving beyond a doubt that the dolphins had indeed moved the human out of the reality of their disorder into a reality free of their disorder when the switches were turned ON in the swimmers.

It would take another ten years of research before we would be able to develop Cranial Dynamics™ Technology, a process that is able to layer more harmonics into each frequency and encode them onto a CD disk creating what would be known as BYONETICS. We would be able to move anyone out of the reality of any mental, physical, or emotional disorder into an area of reality free from this pain and suffering.

CHAPTER TEN

Huff Puff
Blow Our House Down Out
Of Here

ANDREW MOVED US TO ARIZONA

After the dolphin research was completed, I took a year off to assimilate all the material accumulated, form an overall view, and once again, decide what the next step would be. As always, the answer was soon in coming.

In August of 1992 the Hurricane Center was reporting that Tropical Storm Andrew had been upgraded to hurricane status and would hit the Florida Keys with Class Five force. Class Five force can only be understood by viewing the comic Gallagher when he smashes a tomato with a sledge hammer. The exodus out of the Keys was much like the scene depicted in the movie *Jaws*, people frantically packing those things that they couldn't live without, mainly T.V. sets, computers and family albums, joining the million plus people on the only highway leaving the Keys and hoping that their back tires crossed over into Miami before Hurricane Andrew closed its jaws and bit the islands in two.

I was busy doing all those things that one does in preparing a house for a hurricane, lighting sage and walking inside and outside our home to cleanse it so it would not draw the destructive energy of Andrew to it. We also packed the essentials and headed off the island toward

Disney World for some fun and relaxation while the gods decided whether they were going to blow our house to the other side of Cuba. I will never forget the feeling of looking at our house for possibly the last time and not knowing whether we would come back to our home or a stack of kindling wood.

All those who left the Keys and migrated into Miami with friends and relatives to escape the wrath of Andrew had a big surprise on the morning that Andrew came onshore. Instead of making a beeline to the Keys, Andrew veered back to the north and hit smack dab in the middle of South Miami. The devastation brought about by the presence of Andrew would have conjured up a deja·vu experience from the survivors of Nagisaki, Japan, after we dropped the atom bomb on them. Close to 200,000 people were displaced. Insurance companies were filing for bankruptcy instead of "lending a helping hand." The government agencies sent in to manage the catastrophe seemed to be adding to the problem more then they were able to solve it. By the time it was over, all the government could do was to give each homeowner just enough money to leave town. Unfortunately, the insurance companies had beat them to it, and with not enough money to rebuild, families had to seek shelter elsewhere. This is when the banks stepped in, foreclosed, and rebuilt new communities with higher price tags, and of course, larger insurance premiums. The American Way!

As for us, the only effect we had from the storm was a missing vent cover on the roof. I know you must be asking yourself whether the burning of the sage saved the Keys from being hit by Andrew. I can only say that results are everything!

With so many people displaced, many families headed to the Keys, which created overcrowding there. Most affected were the schools. Classes doubled in size from 25 to 50 students, with new classrooms being created in the hallways. Also a slew of out-of-state workers came to take advantage of all the new construction and to steal anything that wasn't tied down. I felt it was time to seek greener pastures. A solution came in the form of a visit to the countries of England and France.

During the year I took off to ponder our research with dolphins, I had the opportunity to do a lecture series in England and France. Attending those lectures at different times were representatives from the National Health Organizations of both countries. France (with the highest health cost per capita) and England (running a close second) were looking for ways to reduce the cost of providing health services. Both thought that if people were taught to maintain their well being, then they would spend less time needing health services thus reducing cost, a novel idea at best.

After my return to the States, I received an invitation to speak with these health representatives to see if I would be interested in creating a model, one that would employ those areas of our research that most empowered the individual to take the responsibility to manage his/her own health. I took on the challenge, but I knew that society as a whole would rather burn the candle at both ends and then take an antacid when the fire hit their stomach.

Looking for greener pastures to escape future hurricanes, I began to look at different cities that would offer a good cross section of individuals who could embrace the idea of preventative medicine and be a community where my family could thrive. Through a series of events that brought the right people together, at the right time, I finally decided to move my family to, of all places, the southwest part of the United States. During the winter months the population seems to double in size to accomodate all those who come to enjoy the warm winter days in an effort to extend and enhance their life force. I met with city fathers, local health officials, and citizen groups, and they all embraced the idea of creating a community-based center that would practice the art of self discovery and maintenance of the spiritual and physical body. We arrived to begin the creation of our community center. As luck would have it, the gods had other plans.

THE CATERPILLAR SPROUTS WINGS

Twenty Years
It Took To Spell Lama
Now One

The New Year had just been celebrated with new friends and old acquaintances. In this case the old acquaintances turned out to be the Lamas of the Tje Jan. Their energy was present to bring full circle over twenty years of spiritual training and move me to the next level of my service, but not before the powers that be would want to kill the messenger.

I was up late. My wife Susan was asleep on the couch. She was soon to give birth to our daughter, Christina. Michael, who became a part of my life when I married Susan, was her son. He was safe and secure in his own bed. He was six years old at this time. I was going over in my mind, while sitting at the kitchen table, different locations for the Health Center when I felt a strong presence of energy emanating from the hallway. I pushed the chair back, stood up, and turned toward the hallway. There before me as I came into the hallway, was this glowing, pulsating, presence of energy.

"Good evening Jean. We haven't been in front of each other for some time," said the Lama.

"It has been awhile," I said. "I have missed your visits."

As a side note, my prior visits with the Lamas had been before I had married Susan. Although she knew about my association with "some lamas" it hadn't been necessary to reveal to her how the Lamas travel through time and space and land in front of me in a ball of energy. You have to be at a certain vibration of energy to see the Lamas in the first place, and Susan didn't have this advantage.

"Jean," said the Lama. "we believe that from our first life to now, we are created from a force that when moved gives birth to all things. This God Force is perfect in nature, and as such, integrates this perfection into everything it creates. Spiritual transformation is the process of remembering whom we have always been every time this perfection is given birth. Meditation releases every negative memory that has kept us separated from the manifestation of this perfection. With every negative memory that is released through meditation, the energy that held that memory is given back to the spiritual body to once again manifest mental, physical, and emotional abundance.

“Every time this transformation takes place, the soul enacts visions of when that perfection was last experienced. In your case, Jean, your soul keeps playing out visions of when you were the Oracle for His Holiness ZshonZshneh, some 26,000 years ago. You are now going to commence your next Intiation. It is here that we are going to open up your physical body to receive the spiritual manifestation of His Holiness’s energy, and within this energy, will His voice become yours."

"I know that all of my training has been to prepare me for this transformation, but unfortunately, I don't have a sense of who His Holiness is."

"Jean, Tje Jan means 'the essence from within.' This philosophy concerns itself with the emergance of an Oracle whose voice will move us out of darkness into Light.

"Over 26,000 years the earth moves through seven levels of regeneration. Remember! Gravity is present not so much to keep us from floating away from earth as much as to press us into the earth so we can receive its vibrations or resonance value. In other words, as the earth vibrates so do we. The earth begins to vibrate and moves itself and its inhabitants into spiritual healing. Once complete, the earth then increases its vibration and heals itself and us cellularly. Then the earth establishes longevity while defining the meditative state that will address physical and emotional pain. As each regenerative cycle is completed, the resonant value of the earth's energy increases so that our awareness of a twenty-four hour cycle is reduced by one hour increments. For example, when the earth completed its first regenerative cycle of spiritual healing, we sensed 24 hours as being 23 hours. This accounts for our sense of time passing faster and faster with each vibrational movement in the earth.

"At this time the earth is seeking physical balance. We see it in extreme weather changes from hot to cold to rain to drought to an increase in earthquakes and hurricanes. Our own physical nature seems to be following the same changing paths. Over population is physically wearing us all down with greater needs and less resources to draw from. In the year 2009 the earth will increase its resonant value and move itself and us into the reality that seeks peace, free of stress and anxiety. By this time 24 hours will seem like 18 hours in our reality. Then on the 21st of December in the year 2012, the earth will complete its 26,000 year cycle of regeneration and begin the process all over again. If our reason for coming back time and again is to resolve conflicts that our ego keeps separating us from in an effort to protect us from the fear of rejection and inadequacy, then it is most important for us to find a way to wipe our karmic slate clean or the next 26,000 year cycle will keep us in Purgatory where darkness overcomes the Light.

"There is an Oracle that appears at the end of the earth's regenerative cycle to help in this transformational process. The Oracle's duty is to connect with the collective consciousness of the six billion plus people on the earth in such a way as to create harmony, balance, and peace, through the perfection of love and abundance without passing judgment.

"This Oracle has always been the voice for the spiritual entity known as His Holiness ZshonZshneh, Seventh Lama of the Tje Jan, Protector of the Mandala of the Soul of the Universe. Since this spiritual entity only appears at the end of the 26,000 year cycle of the earth's regenerational cycle, he is not known to any spiritual masters on this earth's plane.

"Jean, we know that you question every day our very existence and your role in all of this. You have always spoken of feeling that you were the guardian for a much larger force, not knowing, of course, that this force was, in reality, you.

"Jean, it is now time for you to become this force and manifest your destiny as the Oracle for His Holiness ZshonZshneh."

During this final transformation, the Lamas provided me with a person who would serve as a witness to acknowledge the transformations that would spiritually turn me from a caterpillar into a butterfly.

I was fortunate to live close to a special canyon area that for centuries has always been used to initiate and accelerate spiritual transformations. Early morning walks with my witness brought about visions of other worlds whose very energy seemed to integrate into my being and join His Holiness's voice with mine.

His Holiness's energy was so strong that when it vibrated through me I would literally shake, much like those times when He visited me as a baby. His voice would scream through my vocal cords and shoot from my mouth in bolts of red lightning. I would yell out at the top of my lungs the Astral Projection Meditation that connects His Holiness's energy to that of the collective consciousness of the six billion plus inhabitants of the earth.

His Holiness cannot sit down with each of the six billion plus people who inhabit this earth and convince them that they, in some way shape or form, are participating in the destruction of our planet. This would require judgment on His part, and that would only bring about more violence. What He can do instead is to use my voice to recite this meditation and project its energy of harmony, balance, and peace through the perfection of love and abundance to each person, thus changing them from the inside out. Eventually this presence of peace welling up inside them will help resolve their conflicts from a negative presence to a positive source of abundance that they can redirect back into the earth, thus saving us from living out 26,000 years in darkness.

On the 31st of January, 1995, I became the Oracle for His Holiness ZshonZshneh, Seventh Lama of the Tje Jan. It was also on this date that the authorities charged me with practicing medicine without a license.

Once again I would have to stand up to my values and integrity to pass yet another Initiation.

THE DOCTOR TAKES IT PERSONALLY

Doctors Heal
The Sick Until They're Out
Of Money

Evidently the complaint came from a particular doctor who had been treating a client with rheumatoid arthritis. Every week for over twenty years, this doctor had been injecting 24K gold solution into the affected joints of this patient. This solution served as a lubricant so there would be less friction when moving. The joke between this doctor and his patient was that when she died he was going to mine her for all the gold she had in her. Instead of getting better over time, her condition was becoming worse. She decided to end these expensive treatments and seek other avenues.

Before we would agree to take on any particular disorder in which the medical profession has ceased to be effective in treating, we required the attending physician to sign off, thus freeing the patient to work with us. After each session the client would be required to sign their Meta Analysis that measured their "before" and "after" response to their treatment, designating that they understood that our services were not provided under any medical authority of license. When this particular client told her doctor with whom she had been friends for so long that she wanted to try brainwave therapy, he turned and walked away without saying a word, leaving her standing alone in his office. The client felt betrayed by her friend. She believed that his friendship with her was based more on the revenue he received from his expensive gold treatments instead of a genuine concern for her well being.

Over a particular period of time of using brainwave therapy, this client was able to move out of the reality that held her arthritis into a reality that was free of the disorder. She began to enjoy a physical regeneration that reduced the negative effects of her condition. Evidently word got back to her doctor of her success, and soon after, he chose to come after me.

The client felt even more violated by her doctor, since he was attacking the very source of her recovery.

As you can well imagine, my wife Susan was going crazy. She was experiencing deep depression after the birth of our daughter Christina, which made it that much more difficult for her to address the needs of what was now “her son” Michael. Her ego had completely separated her from the source of her feelings of rejection and inadequacy which was me. I was telling my brain, every minute of every hour, to change this energy from a negative to a positive source of abundance that would give me the power to stand up for my values and integrity and end this assault on me and my family. I remember one afternoon laying down in an effort to recover from my mental, physical, and emotional exhaustion when a high pitched tone began to sound in my ears. Then a voice said, "Jean, you are almost there."

"I'm almost where?" I said in somewhat of a hazy, dreamlike state.

"You have reset enough energy from a negative to a positive source of abundance to bring this adventure to a close."

"Adventure?" I said with a bark of indignation. "Adventure? I have proven myself for over twenty years, and now, at the time that I have become an Oracle, I am accused with doing something more right than wrong. I've got to tell you, I've had about as much fun as I can possibly stand."

"Jean, the voice inside your mind is not the voice of the Lamas but mine, the voice of ZshonZshneh. It is I who have chosen you to represent me to the world. You have to know that there are going to be many self professed healers who are going to be threatened by your presence. Why would they act any other way? They are too busy healing others to have time to address their own conflicts, and when you confront them, they are going to attack. Your ability to take the negative energy and change it, moment by moment, into a positive force that is working for you is going to be your saving grace. You don't have to reset 51% of the negative energy present. You only have to reset 16%. One and six add up to seven. Seven is the transformational number between the physical and spiritual bodies. Only 16% of the population had to be convinced that your country was wrong to be in Vietnam. Once that 16% was reset from a negative to a positive force, then the other 84% had to follow. And it is the same here. 16% has been reset. Every moment you have changed the energy emitting from those who are persecuting you to a positive force without making a judgment as to why they are wrong. If you had judged their wrong doing, you would have to resolve the conflict that caused this doctor to attack you in an effort to cover up his own inadequacies, and then this ordeal would never end until you resolved your conflict with him. And as we know, that could take forever."

"Are you telling me that this complaint is going to be dropped?" My voice was filled with doubt.

"I am saying that someone unknown to you is going to appear with the necessary resources to resolve this conflict so you and your family can can be whole again."

A friend told my story over dinner to some friends who were visiting. A woman who was one of his guests had also been attacked by individuals who were afraid of the message she was giving in her lectures, and through the help of others, she prevailed. In an effort to bring things full circle, she and her husband got involved and within a two week period of time, the complaint had been resolved to the satisfaction of all concerned. Since this incident I have been attacked again and again by those who want to kill the messenger. I have prevailed every time due to my ability to continually tell my brain, "Change it to a positive." Remember! The brain doesn't have a mind of its own. It only has my voice to direct it. Once I took the responsibility to be the Master of the Moment and maintain a positive presence in the "Now," did I have dominion over my life as a spiritual being in a physical body.

EMERGENCE OF THE ORACLE

Oracle Voice
Reset Course Karmic Freedom
No Remorse

As an Oracle I am able to go back into the cellular memory of any life force and find the conflict that over time has manifested into disorder and change that energy from a negative to a positive force. This disorder can be felt within the person as mental, physical, or emotional pain, or within countries whose greed has brought about war, or within our leaders where corporate support has robbed them of their ability to serve the very people that elected them.

I have created an organization known as THEE FORCE. THEE FORCE is dedicated to bringing back mental clarity, physical vitality, emotional balance, and financial prosperity to support this spiritual wellness into all the families of the world through non-violence.

As the Lamas said, we cannot individually sit down with six billion plus people who inhabit this earth and convince them that we are destroying this planet, but we can use each of the seven colors to astral project harmony, balance, and peace through the perfection of love and abundance to 16% of this collective. Once our unconditional gift is received, then this harmony, balance, and peace will prevail in their thoughts and actions, and we will move out of darkness into Light.

THE ORACLE GOES TO WORK

Millennium Y2K
Are We Going To Perish
Not yet

Over the millennium the Lamas invited me to address the growing concern by world leaders that Pakistan was about to drop a neutron bomb on India. I went back into the cellular memory of Pakistan and found a conflict that had been festering since 1959, when through the efforts of Gandhi, British rule ended, and what was one country before was divided into Pakistan and India. Pakistan always felt that India was poking them with the short end of the stick, and that by dropping the bomb, Pakistan would regain its prominence over India. Thirty-six hours after I changed this energy from a negative to a positive force, Pakistan moved out of darkness into the Light, and this most dangerous situation was diffused.

North Korea, considered to be a rogue nation, was creating fear over its ability to aim its nuclear missiles at world capitals. I provided an oracle that pinpointed the exact time when conflicts occurred that caused North Korea to make such choices. Within 48 hours after I reset this energy to a positive force for change, North Korea unexpectantly opened up the 38th Parallel for the first time in 55 years and began the reuniting of North and South Korea.

During an unprecedented seven day visit by Secretary of State Madeline Albright, Kim Jong II, the President of

North Korea, promised to dismantle their nuclear weapons. Since then the President of South Korea, Kim Dae-jung, has won the Nobel Peace Prize for his "Sunshine Policy" of engaging North Korea in peace negotiations.

The Lamas felt it necessary to enlist my services during the Gore-Bush Presidential election. After the oracle defined a conflict in representation between big business and the common man, I stepped in and reset the energy to a positive force, and the United States had its own electoral revolution. Citizens were finally realizing that their vote did count.

After oracles were completed on the country of Chile , it began to challenge its own political process. Mexico broke away from a totalitarian government and elected a new president that represents the poor more than the rich. Yugoslavia finally removed their president who believed in "ethnic cleansing." Russia is freeing itself of old Soviet roots whose policies did little to improve the welfare of its people.

By the time the year 2000 had ended, I had completed an oracle and reset the energy of some 162 countries from a negative to a positive force for change.

In 2001 I committed my time to completing oracles for all the leaders of these countries. What was most interesting was that the conflict of every leader centered around their profession as a leader, ruler, or king, and all of them were affected financially more than emotionally with the fear of inadequacy in doing their job correctly. No wonder the world is in the mess it is in where, in the 20th

Century alone, over 100,000 million people have been killed to justify the actions of these so called leaders. I have also done oracles for the representatives of our own political parties here in the United States and the President and his cabinet. I have completed oracles for all those individuals whose voice as an actor, professional athelete, or author, touch the collective with their energy.

For those who experience pain and suffering, I offer my services as an oracle to go back into their cellular memories and reset any conflicts. This is by far the most important thing to do when addressing any disorder, for if you don't resolve the conflict that created the disorder in the first place, it won't matter what modality you use to treat it, the disorder will keep reappearing.

The year 2002 was dedicated to developing a less expensive way of delivering the healing frequencies of the dolphins to those sufferers who have exhausted all the medical benefits available to them and still want another chance at life.

By going to www•theeforce•org you can learn about BYONETICS and find out how we have been successful in receiving a provisional patent on Cranial Dynamics™ Technology. This technology encodes layers of harmonic frequencies onto a CD disk. By listening to this amazing CD while going to sleep, the sufferer has the opportunity to move out of the reality of his disorder into a reality of harmony, balance, and peace. Now the individual can move down to a weight that supports better sleep, less depression and anxiety, access to more memory, superlearning, reduced signs of aging, less need to use addictive substances like cigarettes with no weight gain, while addressing overall stress..

Once BYONETICS has been employed, we offer the opportunity for our clients to come down to the islands of the Florida Keys to swim with our beloved dolphins and manifest their destiny as spiritual beings in physical bodies in harmony, balance, and peace through the perfection of love and abundance, and move out of darkness into Light.

I have also provided a permanent home for the Mandala of the Soul of the Universe here at our gallery in the Florida Keys. People come from around the world to stand in front of the Mandala and receive its healing energies.

A typical day at our spiritual retreat starts out on the beach with the Thousand Breaths of the Lotus. This ancient breathing exercise connects us to the Universal Mind Substance where we receive the perfection that we will astral project to all the inhabitants of the earth. I then begin chanting the Meditation of the Lamas. This meditation frees us of the physical plane so we can spiritually ascend to a point where we can project this harmony, balance, and peace to all the inhabitants of the world. Once complete we move into the graceful movements of Tai Chi and finish with the Lamas' Yoga. We then enjoy a light breakfast and get back together mid-morning in front of the Mandala so we can access the Other Side and address any conflicts that are manifesting into disorder within the individual, their association with their mate, family, friends, or profession. In our afternoon session we experience BYONETICS technology by listening to the rejuvenation frequencies that are on this amazing CD. This prepares us for our swim with the dolphins. I provide a dolphin orientation. This is where I make the swimmers familar with the super powers that the dolphin possesses and how the dolphins will use this power to move us into realities where success is experienced free of pain and suffering.One's experience with the dolphins is so mentally, physically, and emotionally, altering that a time is provided to just lie down with the BYONETICS CD and merge into our spiritual essence. Evening dinner is filled with gaiety. A lot has happened in such a short period of time that there is a need to voice this energy in the form of questions that lead to discussions that come full circle with an new understanding of who were are as a spiritual being in this physical body.

Each day is filled with the same elements of meditation and mental and physical exercise that prepare us for our experience with the dolphins that will expand our spiritual dynamic.

There are some who come to visit us for just a day; then there are those who use each day that they are here with us and the dolphins to keep pushing the envelope of their human existence to new heights of spiritual awakening.

Whatever your mental, physical, and/or emotional needs are, we are Thee Force in providing you with mental clarity, physical vitality, and emotional balance that brings you full circle spiritually in a way that is financially affordable.

We can be reached by mail at:

Thee Force
PO Box 283
Tavernier Island, FL. 33070

1.800.280.2802

info@theeforce.org

Our website addresses are:

www.theeforce.org
or
www.cranialdynamics.net

We look forward to being of service.

I respectfully remain,

Jean Charles Genet

Dolphin Oracle
One In The Same With
Their Voice

ACKNOWLEDGEMENTS

I didn't want to miss the opportunity to express my sincere apreciation to certain individuals who have been instrumental in bringing *Dolphin & The Oracle* to completion.

First of all, I want to thank a multitude of individuals (You know who you are.) who sought every possible way to verify times, dates, and happenings of my final mission where I crashed in the helicopter, my rehabilitation files, and my work with NASA, but none seems to exist. To be fair the government withholds any information from general circulation for reasons of national security when that activity is done in places outside the accepted jurisdiction.

Also there are always "well meaning" individuals who are continually wanting to protect their spiritual and/or educational domain by attacking anyone who challenges accepted views of practice and thought. The Lamas believe that I should be complimented by their need to attack me since I evidently threaten them not so much by my research, but more so for the positive results clients have received. I have to admit that there are certain aspects of my story that stretch the envelope of believability. Hell, I still have a hard time adjusting to the fact that my experiences with the Lamas are real. And if I have a hard time with all of this, where does this leave you, the reader? But you have to admit that it is an incredible story providing invaluable insight into the human condition. If after all this you still have doubts, then please look upon this work as fiction...*the assumption of a possible truth.*

I want to thank Kerry Hoffman for providing a style and pace to the written word that I found invaluable as I took his lead.

I want to thank Barbara Lord, Angela Karlson, and Trish Pleasant for continually editing my writing while still keeping my personality intact.

The Lamas believe that the greatest thing any one person can do is continually earn the right to have something greater happen to them spiritually so it can be manifested into a physical form of service. The Lamas have been of great service to me and all those they serve with the presence of their energy.

Finally, I want to acknowledge all of my soul mates. These are individuals who challenge who I am, what I stand for and how that can be of service to others. If I have been your son, your brother, your lover, your mate, your father, your friend, your associate, your teacher, your advisor or your enemy, then you qualify as my soul mate, and I thank you with all my heart for being part of an incredible journey where values and integrity always serve as the final test.

Notes

Notes

Notes

Notes

Notes